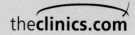

ULTRASOUND CLINICS

Pediatric Ultrasound

Guest Editor
BRIAN D. COLEY, MD

Intraoperative Ultrasonography of the Abdomen

Guest Editors
JONATHAN B. KRUSKAL, MD, PhD
ROBERT A. KANE, MD

July 2006 • Volume 1 • Number 3

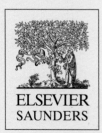

ELSEVIER
SAUNDERS

An imprint of Elsevier, Inc
PHILADELPHIA LONDON TORONTO MONTREAL SYDNEY TOKYO

W.B. SAUNDERS COMPANY
A Division of Elsevier Inc.

1600 John F. Kennedy Boulevard • Suite 1800 • Philadelphia, Pennsylvania 19103-2899

http://www.theclinics.com

ULTRASOUND CLINICS Volume 1, Number 3
July 2006 ISSN 1556-858X, ISBN 1-4160-3731-4

Editor: Barton Dudlick

Reprints: For copies of 100 or more, of articles in this publication, please contact the Commercial Reprints Department, Elsevier Inc., 360 Park Avenue South, New York, New York 10010-1710. Tel.: (+1) 212-633-3813; Fax: (+1) 212-462-1935 Email: reprints@elsevier.com

The ideas and opinions expressed in *Ultrasound Clinics* do not necessarily reflect those of the Publisher. The Publisher does not assume any responsibility for any injury and/or damage to persons or property arising out of or related to any use of the material contained in this periodical. The reader is advised to check the appropriate medical literature and the product information currently provided by the manufacturer of each drug to be administered to verify the dosage, the method and duration of administration, or contraindications. It is the responsibility of the treating physician or other health care professional, relying on independent experience and knowledge of the patient, to determine drug dosages and the best treatment for the patient. Mention of any product in this issue should not be construed as endorsement by the contributors, editors, or the Publisher of the product or manufacturers' claims.

Ultrasound Clinics (ISSN 1556-858X) is published quarterly by W.B. Saunders, 360 Park Avenue South, New York, NY 10010-1710. Months of publication are January, April, July, and October. Business and editorial offices: 1600 John F. Kennedy Boulevard, Suite 1800, Philadelphia, Pennsylvania 19103-2899. Accounting and circulation offices: 6277 Sea Harbor Drive, Orlando, FL 32887-4800. Periodicals postage paid at New York NY, and additional mailing offices. Subscription prices are USD 150 per year for US individuals, USD 210 per year for US institutions, USD 75 per year for US students and residents, USD 170 per year for Canadian individuals, USD 200 per year for Canadian institutions, USD 170 per year for international individuals, USD 230 per year for international institutions, and USD 85 per year for Canadian and foreign students/residents. To receive student/resident rate, orders must be accompanied by name of affiliated institution, date of term, and the signature of program/residency coordinator on institution letterhead. Orders will be billed at individual rate until proof of status is received. Foreign air speed delivery is included in all Clinics subscription prices. All prices are subject to change without notice. **POSTMASTER:** Send address changes to *Ultrasound Clinics*, Elsevier Periodicals Customer Service, 6277 Sea Harbor Drive, Orlando, FL 32887-4800. **Customer Service: 1-800-654-2452 (US). From outside of the US, call (+1) 407-345-4000.**

Printed in the United States of America.

PEDIATRIC ULTRASOUND INTRAOPERATIVE ULTRASONOGRAPHY OF THE ABDOMEN

ROBERT A. KANE, MD, FACR
Professor of Radiology, Harvard Medical
School; and Co-Chief of Ultrasound,
Department of Radiology, Beth Israel Deaconess
Medical Center, Boston, Massachusetts

JONATHAN B. KRUSKAL, MD, PhD
Associate Professor of Radiology, Harvard Medical
School; Chief, Abdominal Imaging, Department
of Radiology, Beth Israel Deaconess Medical
Center, Boston, Massachusetts

MICHAEL RICCABONA, MD
Professor, Department of Radiology, Division of
Pediatric Radiology, University Hospital, Graz,
Austria

SABAH SERVAES, MD
Assistant Professor Radiology, The Children's
Hospital of Philadelphia, Philadelphia, Pennsylvania

MARILYN J. SIEGEL, MD
Professor of Radiology and Pediatrics,
Mallinckrodt Institute of Radiology, Washington
University School of Medicine, St. Louis,
Missouri

BETTINA SIEWERT, MD
Staff Radiologist, Department of Radiology,
Beth Israel Deaconess Medical Center,
and Assistant Professor of Radiology,
Harvard Medical School, Boston,
Massachusetts

JACOB SOSNA, MD
Department of Radiology, Beth Israel
Deaconess Medical Center,
Harvard Medical School, Boston,
Massachusetts; Department of Radiology,
Hadassah-Hebrew University Medical Center,
Jerusalem, Israel

PETER J. STROUSE, MD
Associate Professor, Section of Pediatric Radiology,
C.S. Mott Children's Hospital, Department of
Radiology, University of Michigan Health System,
Ann Arbor, Michigan

PEDIATRIC ULTRASOUND
INTRAOPERATIVE ULTRASONOGRAPHY
OF THE ABDOMEN

Volume 1 · Number 3 · July 2006

Contents

that cannot be sufficiently diagnosed by clinical, laboratory, and imaging findings. Finally, US offers treatment options by guiding interventions, such as percutaneous nephrostomy. Only rarely are additional imaging modalities such as MR imaging, fluoroscopy, or scintigraphy indicated, usually for completing the diagnostic work-up of a condition after stabilizing the acute situation.

Sonographic Evaluation of the Child with Lower Abdominal or Pelvic Pain   471

Peter J. Strouse

At many centers, CT has become the primary imaging modality for children who have abdominal pain. CT, however, delivers a substantial radiation dose, which is of particular concern in the pediatric patient. In contrast, sonography does not expose the patient to ionizing radiation. Properly performed, sonography is capable of providing useful diagnostic information in the child who has lower abdominal or pelvic pain. In many children and with many disorders, sonography proves to be the only imaging modality that may be required. In this article, the usefulness of sonography in evaluating disorders producing lower abdominal or pelvic pain in a child is reviewed.

The Acute Pediatric Scrotum   485

Brian D. Coley

Proper evaluation of the acute scrotum starts with a history and physical examination by an experienced clinician. The true nature of the underlying condition producing scrotal pain is not always clear, however. Ultrasound is the single most useful imaging tool for imaging the scrotum. Properly performed and interpreted, ultrasound provides very high sensitivity and specificity for acute scrotal conditions. Understanding the characteristic sonographic features of the conditions producing acute scrotal pain in children allows the examining physician to make more accurate and confident diagnoses. It is hoped that this article helps promote this understanding.

The Painful Extremity   497

Sabah Servaes and Richard Bellah

As technologic improvements continue, imaging increasingly becomes more powerful and faster, having an impact on choices of modality and technique. Sonography's role in musculoskeletal imaging of pediatric patients is steadfast but evolving. The lack of radiation, ease of examination, lower cost, and dynamic nature of the sonographic examination are factors contributing to its central role in imaging in general, and its ability to demonstrate cartilaginous and soft tissue structures in patients who are skeletally immature contributes to its importance in pediatric musculoskeletal imaging in particular.

Preface: Intraoperative Ultrasonography of the Abdomen   509

Jonathan B. Kruskal and Robert A. Kane

Intraoperative Ultrasonography of the Liver: Why, When, and How?   511

Liat Appelbaum, Jonathan B. Kruskal, Jacob Sosna, and Robert A. Kane

Intraoperative ultrasonography (IOUS) of the liver is used with increasing frequency as an adjunct to surgical planning. It provides interactive, vital, real-time information to surgeons during the procedure and has an impact on the clinical decision-making process. IOUS of the liver has many applications, including tumor staging, metastatic surveys, guidance for metastasectomy and the various tumor ablation procedures, documentation of vessel patency, evaluation of intrahepatic biliary disease, and guidance for whole organ or split liver transplantation.

Intraoperative ultrasonography is an important adjunct to surgical procedures involving the intra- and extrahepatic biliary system. The technique adds to characterization of disease entities and is helpful particularly in establishing the full extent of a disease process that often is underestimated by preoperative imaging studies. It can have, therefore, a major impact on surgical planning and tumor staging.

Intraoperative ultrasound of the pancreas is an invaluable adjunct to surgeons and has a wide spectrum of diagnostic usefulness in confirming suspected pathology, identifying occult pathology, and guiding several intraoperative procedures. In some conditions, such as the operative management of neuroendocrine tumors, its use reflects standard of care and serves as a gold standard. This review describes its application across the spectrum of pancreatic disease, ranging from neoplastic to inflammatory, and encompassing acute and chronic pathology. Essential facts and useful tips and techniques are described.

In parallel with the increasing move from open surgical procedures to laparoscopic approaches, laparoscopic ultrasound (LUS) is being used with increasing frequency to image normal structures and intra-abdominal pathology. Special transducers and scanning techniques are required to perform LUS with a different set of considerations. Within the spectrum of LUS applications, LUS is used to complement laparoscopy for oncology staging, to facilitate an array of surgical procedures, and to guide laparoscopic biopsies.

ULTRASOUND CLINICS JULY 2006

GOAL STATEMENT

The goal of the *Ultrasound Clinics* is to keep practicing radiologists and radiology residents up to date with current clinical practice in ultrasound by providing timely articles reviewing the state-of-the-art in patient care.

ACCREDITATION

The *Ultrasound Clinics* is planned and implemented in accordance with the Essential Areas and Policies of the Accreditation Council for Continuing Medical Education (ACCME) through the joint sponsorship of the University of Virginia School of Medicine and Elsevier. The University of Virginia School of Medicine is accredited by the ACCME to provide continuing medical education for physicians.

The University of Virginia School of Medicine designates this educational activity for a maximum of 15 *AMA PRA Category 1 Credits™*. Physicians should only claim credit commensurate with the extent of their participation in the activity.

The American Medical Association has determined that physicians not licensed in the US who participate in this CME activity are eligible for 15 *AMA PRA Category 1 Credits™*.

Category 1 credit can be earned by reading the text material, taking the CME examination online at http://www.theclinics.com/home/cme, and completing the evaluation. After taking the test, you will be required to review any and all incorrect answers. Following completion of the test and evaluation, your credit will be awarded and you may print your certificate.

FACULTY DISCLOSURE/CONFLICT OF INTEREST

The University of Virginia School of Medicine, as an ACCME accredited provider, endorses and strives to comply with the Accreditation Council for Continuing Medical Education (ACCME) Standards of Commercial Support, Commonwealth of Virginia statutes, University of Virginia policies and procedures, and associated federal and private regulations and guidelines on the need for disclosure and monitoring of proprietary and financial interests that may affect the scientific integrity and balance of content delivered in continuing medical education activities under our auspices.

The University of Virginia School of Medicine requires that all CME activities accredited through this institution be developed independently and be scientifically rigorous, balanced and objective in the presentation/discussion of its content, theories and practices.

All authors/editors participating in an accredited CME activity are expected to disclose to the readers relevant financial relationships with commercial entities occurring within the past 12 months (such as grants or research support, employee, consultant, stock holder, member of speakers bureau, etc.). The University of Virginia School of Medicine will employ appropriate mechanisms to resolve potential conflicts of interest to maintain the standards of fair and balanced education to the reader. Questions about specific strategies can be directed to the Office of Continuing Medical Education, University of Virginia School of Medicine, Charlottesville, Virginia.

The authors/editors listed below have identified no professional or financial affiliations for themselves or their spouse/partner:
Liat Appelbaum, MD; Richard Bellah, MD; Darren D. Brennan, MD; Brian D. Coley, MD; Barton Dudlick, Acquisitions Editor; Suvranu Ganguli, MD; Zoltan Harkanyi, MD, PhD; Robert A. Kane, MD, FACR; Jonathan B. Kruskal, MD, PhD; Sabah Servaes, MD; Bettina Siewert, MD; Jacob Sosna, MD; and, Peter J. Strouse, MD.

The authors/editors listed below have identified the following professional or financial affiliations for themselves or their spouse/partner:
Michael Riccabona, MD has ongoing research and counseling cooperation on US and MRI with Siemens, and Acuson, and is on the Advisory Board for 3DUS (Kretz / General Electrics).
Marilyn J. Siegel, MD is on the speaker's bureau for Siemens Medical Solutions and Phillips Medical.

Disclosure of Discussion of non-FDA approved uses for pharmaceutical products and/or medical devices:
The University of Virginia School of Medicine, as an ACCME provider, requires that all faculty presenters identify and disclose any "off label" uses for pharmaceutical and medical device products. The University of Virginia School of Medicine recommends that each physician fully review all the available data on new products or procedures prior to instituting them with patients.

TO ENROLL

To enroll in the *Ultrasound Clinics* Continuing Medical Education program, call customer service at **1-800-654-2452** or visit us online at www.theclinics.com/home/cme. The CME program is available to subscribers for an additional fee *of* $205.00.

ULTRASOUND
CLINICS

Ultrasound Clin 1 (2006) xi

Preface

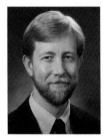

Brian D. Coley, MD
Guest Editor

Brian D. Coley, MD
Department of Radiology
Columbus Children's Hospital
700 Children's Drive
Columbus, OH 43205, USA

E-mail address:
bcoley@chi.osu.edu

This issue of the *Ultrasound Clinics* reviews some of the uses of ultrasound in the pediatric patient. Given their generally smaller size, children are ideal candidates for ultrasound evaluation. In the current imaging environment, MR imaging and CT receive the most interest of all of the modalities, and they are powerful indeed. However, radiologists in North America are finally gaining the awareness of our European colleagues about the potential detrimental effects of diagnostic radiation in the very young, and MR imaging often requires sedation and is not always expediently available. Ultrasound is often underappreciated in the face of these other modalities. Pediatric ultrasound provides detailed anatomic information and is the original multiplanar modality. Doppler studies can add important functional and physiological information. Any imaging modality can only provide the information that you know how to look for, and

you only recognize the conditions that you know. Ultrasound, unfortunately, is often given little weight in current radiology training, is often poorly understood by practicing radiologists, and often relegated to a screening role until the patient can be scheduled for CT or MRI. This is unfortunate. It only takes a little bit of effort to understand ultrasound (even scanning a patient yourself on occasion) to appreciate what real-time gray-scale and Doppler evaluation can show.

The contributing authors bring a wealth of international experience and perspective to pediatric ultrasound. I am grateful to them for their efforts. Thanks are also due to Barton Dudlick and the staff of Elsevier for their expertise and care in production. I hope that the articles presented here interest you, help you to care for the children you encounter, and encourage you to explore and expand the use of ultrasound in your practice.

ultrasound.theclinics.com

doi:10.1016/j.cult.2006.06.001

ULTRASOUND
CLINICS

Ultrasound Clin 1 (2006) 431–441

Jaundice in Infants and Children

Marilyn J. Siegel, MD

- Sonographic examination
- Overview of cholestatic diseases
- Neonatal jaundice
  Biliary atresia
  Neonatal hepatitis syndrome
  Additional imaging studies to
     differentiate atresia and hepatitis
  Alagille syndrome
  Choledochal cyst
- *Spontaneous perforation of the*
     extrahepatic bile ducts
  Inspissated bile syndrome
- Jaundice in older infants and children
  Caroli disease
  Byler disease
  Hepatocellular diseases
  Inflammatory diseases of the biliary ducts
  Biliary tract obstruction
- References

Real-time sonography remains the screening study of choice for the evaluation of jaundice in infants and children and it is an important tool in differentiating between obstructive and nonobstructive causes of jaundice [1,2]. The causes of cholestasis are multiple, but the three major causes are hepatitis, biliary atresia, and choledochal cyst. Other causes include neoplastic processes, cirrhosis, and strictures.

This article reviews the common congenital and acquired causes of jaundice in the pediatric patient and describes the sonographic findings associated with these conditions. The role of correlative imaging studies is also reviewed.

Sonographic examination

The sonographic examination of infants and children who have jaundice includes a detailed examination of the liver, bile ducts, gallbladder, and pancreas. Hepatic size and echotexture should be thoroughly assessed. The right hepatic lobe should extend to or just below the right costal margin in a patient without hyperinflated lungs. The echogenicity of the normal liver is low to medium and homogeneous, and the central portal venous vasculature is easily seen (Fig. 1). In the neonate and young infant, the hepatic parenchyma and renal cortex are equally echogenic. In individuals 6 months of age and older, the liver usually is more echogenic than the kidney. The patency and flow direction of the hepatic vessels should be documented with pulsed and color Doppler interrogation. The liver and adjacent area should also be evaluated for evidence of end-stage liver disease, including collateral channels (varices), hepatofugal flow, and ascites.

The diameter of the common duct should be measured on the sagittal scan to confirm the presence or absence of ductal dilatation. The upper limits of the common duct should not exceed 1 mm in neonates, 2 mm in infants up to 1 year of age, 4 mm in children 1 to 10 years of age, and 6 mm in adolescents and young adults [3]. The distal portion of the common duct is typically larger than the proximal portion. Ductal size may increase by 1 mm or more during deep inspiration and the Valsalva maneuver [4]. The cystic duct in children

Radiology and Pediatrics, Mallinckrodt Institute of Radiology, Washington University School of Medicine, 510 South Kingshighway Boulevard, St. Louis, MO, 63110, USA
E-mail address: siegelm@mir.wustl.edu

1556-858X/06/$ – see front matter © 2006 Elsevier Inc. All rights reserved.
ultrasound.theclinics.com

doi:10.1016/j.cult.2006.05.010

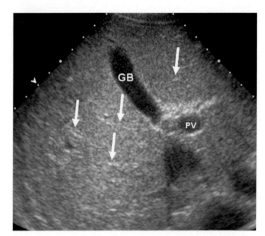

Fig. 1. Normal liver. Transverse sonogram shows homogeneous hepatic parenchyma. The echogenic portal venous vasculature (*arrows*) is easily seen. The gallbladder (GB) is distended and the wall is thin and hyperechoic. PV, portal vein.

is not routinely seen unless it is dilated, and then usually only the distal part of the duct near its insertion into the common bile duct is seen.

Gallbladder size usually can be assessed subjectively, but measurements may be helpful in equivocal cases. The normal gallbladder length is 1.5 to 3.0 cm in neonates and young infants (younger than 1 year old) and the width is approximately 1 cm. In older children and adolescents, gallbladder length is 3 to 8 cm and width is less than 3.5 cm. The wall of the gallbladder should be thin, hyperechoic, and well defined. The upper limits of wall thickness in the fasting state are 3 mm [5].

Feeding of a fatty meal may be helpful in patients who have enlarged gallbladders to assess cystic duct patency. In healthy individuals, maximum emptying of the gallbladder occurs between 45 and 60 minutes after the fatty meal, and the mean volume decreases approximately 60%. Contraction of the gallbladder after a fatty meal supports the diagnosis of a patent cystic duct.

Pancreatic size, echotexture, and ductal size should be evaluated. Pancreatic size increases with increasing age of the child [6]. The mean cross-sectional diameter of the pancreatic head ranges between 1 and 2 cm, the body between 0.6 and 1.1 cm, and the tail between 1 and 2 cm. The normal pancreas is isoechoic or minimally hyperechoic compared with the liver. The cross-sectional diameter of the pancreatic duct should not exceed 1 to 2 mm.

Overview of cholestatic diseases

Causes of cholestasis vary with patient age. For this review, diseases are classified into two main classes:

(1) neonatal and (2) older child and adolescent. In the neonate, biliary atresia, the neonatal hepatitis syndrome, and choledochal cyst are the most common causes of jaundice [7–9]. Other causes include syndromic and nonsyndromic bile duct paucity, inspissated bile syndrome, and spontaneous perforation of the extrahepatic bile duct. In older children, jaundice is most often caused by hepatocellular disease, including hepatitis and cirrhosis. Biliary tract obstruction is a less common cause of childhood jaundice. The possible causes of obstructive jaundice include choledochal cyst, cholangitis, stricture, stones, and neoplasms.

The results of various laboratory tests of liver function, in conjunction with the pertinent historical and physical findings, generally suffice to differentiate between obstructive and nonobstructive causes of jaundice. Imaging examinations are used to confirm the clinical impression. In patients who have obstructive jaundice, these studies may also often show the level and cause of obstruction.

Sonography is the preliminary imaging procedure. If the extrahepatic ducts are well visualized by sonography and are normal in caliber and there is no evidence of intraductal dilatation, further radiologic evaluation is rarely needed. Sonography is supplemented by radionuclide studies using hepatobiliary agents (^{99m}Tc-IDA analogs) when functional information is needed. Hepatobiliary scintigraphy currently is used primarily to confirm suspected diagnoses of choledochal cysts, biliary atresia, and neonatal hepatitis. CT or MR imaging are reserved for cases in which more anatomic detail is needed for surgical planning or the level or cause of obstruction cannot be determined by sonography [10–15].

Neonatal jaundice

Biliary atresia

Biliary atresia is a rare disease with an incidence of 1 in 8,000 to 10,000 live births. It is, however, the single most common cause of neonatal cholestasis, accounting for nearly 90% of the surgical causes and for approximately 40% of all causes of cholestasis [16]. The cause is unclear, but it is believed to be caused by in utero inflammation that results in failure of the remodeling process at the hepatic hilum [7]. Histologically, it is characterized by absence of the extrahepatic bile ducts, proliferation of the small intrahepatic bile ducts, periportal fibrosis, and occasionally multinucleated giant cells. There is a spectrum of changes, depending on the extent of the obliterative process. Complete atresia is present in 75% to 85% of cases. In the remaining cases, there may be patency of the gallbladder and cystic duct or patency of only the gallbladder. Associated anomalies are common (10%–20% of patients) and include choledochal cyst, polysplenia, pre-duodenal portal vein, azygous continuation of the inferior vena cava, diaphragmatic hernia, situs inversus, and hydronephrosis [16–18].

Patients who have biliary atresia and neonatal hepatitis usually present at 1 to 4 weeks of age with jaundice. Distinguishing between neonatal hepatitis and biliary atresia is important, because biliary atresia requires early surgical intervention to prevent biliary cirrhosis, whereas neonatal hepatitis is managed medically. Surgical treatment varies with the level of obstruction [7,8]. When there is extrahepatic biliary obstruction (15%–25% of cases), a direct anastomosis between the patent portion of the extrahepatic bile duct and intestine is performed. When there is intrahepatic biliary atresia, a Kasai hepatoportoenterostomy (anastomosis of a segment of small bowel to the portal region) is performed [7,8,19]. The success rate of the Kasai procedure is inversely proportional to patient age. Bile flow can be re-established in up to 90% of infants who are younger than 2 months of age at the time of hepatoportoenterostomy and in approximately 50% in those who are 2 to 3 months. The success rate decreases to less than 20% when surgery is performed after 90 days of age because of the presence of cirrhosis [7–9]. Liver transplantation is often required in older infants and children who have intrahepatic biliary atresia.

A spectrum of findings may be seen sonographically, reflecting the underlying histology. The liver size and parenchymal echogenicity may be normal or increased [1]. The intrahepatic ducts are typically not dilated. The extrahepatic duct is typically not visualized. A remnant of the extrahepatic duct, however, may be noted in the porta hepatis [20–23]. This remnant appears as a triangular or tubular echogenic structure just superior to the portal vein bifurcation. This finding has been termed the triangular cord sign and correlates with fibrous tissue in the porta hepatis at histologic examination (Fig. 2). The sign is reliable for the diagnosis of extrahepatic biliary atresia and has a specificity approaching 100% and a sensitivity of approximately 85%.

In biliary atresia, the gallbladder is usually small or absent (Fig. 3), although a normal-sized gallbladder may be seen when the atresia is distal to the insertion of the cystic duct (approximately 10% of cases). The finding of a small gallbladder (<1.5 cm in diameter) is nonspecific and may be seen with biliary atresia or neonatal hepatitis. Contractility and changes in gallbladder size after a milk feeding are rare in patients who have biliary atresia (<10% of cases) [24,25].

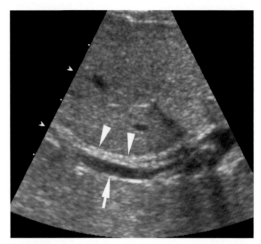

Fig. 2. Biliary atresia, cord sign. Transverse sonogram through the porta hepatis shows an echogenic cord (*arrowheads*) anterior to the portal vein (*arrow*), indicating fibrosis along the course of the common hepatic duct.

Neonatal hepatitis syndrome

The neonatal hepatitis syndrome is the term given to nonspecific hepatic inflammation that develops secondary to several different causes, including infection (cytomegalovirus, herpes simplex, toxoplasmosis, protozoa, syphilis), metabolic defects (alpha 1-antitrypsin deficiency, galactosemia, glycogen storage disease, tyrosinosis), and Alagille syndrome.

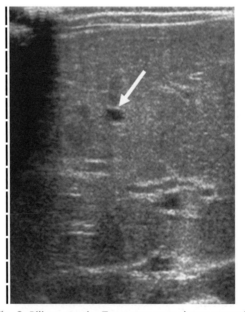

Fig. 3. Biliary atresia. Transverse scan shows normal parenchymal echogenicity. The gallbladder (*arrow*) is small. The common bile duct was not visualized.

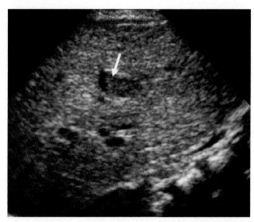

Fig. 4. Neonatal hepatitis. Longitudinal sonogram shows diffusely increased and coarsened echogenicity. The gallbladder is small and filled with sludge (*arrow*).

Histologic examination shows multinucleated giant cells with hepatic parenchymal disruption and little bile within the bile duct canaliculi. Similar to biliary atresia, the cause is believed to be an in utero inflammatory process and the disease process usually manifests with jaundice at 3 to 4 weeks of life.

At sonography, the liver size and echogenicity may be normal or increased, and the biliary ducts are not dilated [1,2] (Fig. 4). The gallbladder may be small, normal, or increased in size. Changes in gallbladder size after a milk feeding can occur in patients who have neonatal hepatitis, reflecting patency of the common hepatic and common bile duct [24].

Additional imaging studies to differentiate atresia and hepatitis

Hepatobiliary scintigraphy

Because the sonographic findings of biliary atresia and hepatitis overlap, hepatobiliary scintigraphy is usually performed to assess the presence or absence of bile excretion into the bowel. Infants who have biliary atresia less than 3 months of age usually show normal hepatic extraction of tracer but no excretion of the radionuclide into the small intestine (Fig. 5A), whereas infants older than 3 months of age show decreased extraction of tracer and no excretion into the bowel. In neonates who have neonatal hepatitis, parenchymal extraction is diminished but there is some excretion into the bowel (Fig. 5B).

The sensitivity and specificity of scintigraphy for the diagnosis of biliary atresia in infants less than 3 months of age is approximately 95% and 80%, respectively. The presence of small bowel activity excludes biliary atresia as the cause of jaundice. Differentiation between biliary atresia and neonatal hepatis is more difficult when there is poor hepatocellular function.

Magnetic resonance imaging

MR cholangiopancreatography may also be useful in assessing the patency of intra- and extrahepatic biliary ducts [10,12]. Complete visualization of the extrahepatic biliary system excludes biliary atresia as the cause of cholestasis [10].

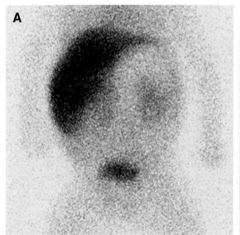
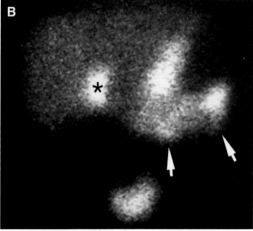

Fig. 5. Hepatobiliary imaging in neonatal jaundice. (*A*) Biliary atresia. Hepatobiliary scan obtained 6 hours after injection of Tc-99m disofenin demonstrates hepatic uptake but absence of excretion into the central bile ducts and intestine. (*B*) Neonatal hepatitis. Hepatobiliary scan obtained 3 hours after injection shows radioactivity in the gallbladder (***) and within bowel (*arrows*). On more delayed images, there was poor clearance of radioactivity from the liver.

Cholangiography

Cholangiography is performed when other clinical or imaging findings suggest the diagnosis of biliary atresia. It may be performed percutaneously, endoscopically, or intraoperatively. Contrast medium is injected into the gallbladder.

Alagille syndrome

Alagille syndrome (also known as arteriohepatic dysplasia) is a hereditary disorder, usually an autosomal dominant trait with variable penetrance [8,26]. A deletion in the short arm of chromosome 20 has been seen in some patients [26]. It is associated with abnormalities of the liver (cholestatic jaundice), heart (most commonly peripheral pulmonic stenosis), skeleton (butterfly vertebrae and hemivertebrae), eye, kidneys, and abnormal facies (frontal bossing, deep-set eyes, bulbous tip of the nose, and pointed chin). The associated findings help to distinguish Alagille syndrome from biliary atresia. Patients typically present with jaundice in the neonatal period. Histologic examination shows paucity and hypoplasia of the interlobular bile ducts. Imaging findings are similar to those described for neonatal hepatitis.

Choledochal cyst

Choledochal cyst is a congenital dilatation of the common bile duct, with 30% of cases found to occur in the first year of life, 50% between 1 and 10 years of age, and 20% in the second decade or later [27]. The classic clinical presentation is jaundice, abdominal pain, and mass, although this triad is present in only 20% to 50% of patients [27]. This abnormality is believed to be the result of an abnormal insertion of the common bile duct into the pancreatic duct, which allows reflux of pancreatic enzymes into the biliary system. This reflux results in a chemical cholangitis, which weakens the walls of the bile duct, eventually leading to ductal dilatation [28].

Four types of choledochal cysts have been described [29]. The type 1 cyst, accounting for 80% to 90% of cases, is subdivided into type 1A, cystic dilatation of the common duct; type 1B, focal segmental common duct dilatation; and type 1C, fusiform dilatation of the common bile duct. The type 2 cyst, accounting for approximately 2% of cases, is a true diverticulum arising from the common duct. The type 3 cyst, accounting for 1% to 5% of cases, is a choledochocele involving only the intraduodenal portion of the duct. The type 4 cyst is subdivided into type 4A, multiple intrahepatic cysts and an extrahepatic cyst, and type 4B, multiple extrahepatic cysts. The type 5 cyst, or Caroli disease, consists of multiple intrahepatic biliary cysts and is considered to be a separate disorder (see later discussion). Choledochal cysts in neonates and young infants may coexist with biliary atresia [17,18].

At sonography, the choledochal cyst appears as a fluid-filled cystic mass in the region of the porta hepatis that is separate from the gallbladder (**Fig. 6**). Intrahepatic biliary duct dilatation is present in approximately half of affected patients and typically is limited to the central portions of the left and right main hepatic ducts. Generalized ductal dilatation, typical of acquired obstruction, is absent. The cysts tend to be smaller and ductal dilatation is absent when there is concomitant biliary atresia [17,18]. Complications associated with choledochal cysts include cholelithiasis, choledocholithiasis, ascending cholangitis, intrahepatic abscesses, biliary cirrhosis, portal hypertension, and hepatobiliary malignancy, usually adenocarcinomas. The risk for malignancy increases with age [27].

When a choledochal cyst is demonstrated sonographically, scintigraphy with hepatobiliary agents is performed to confirm that the cystic mass communicates with the biliary system. Preoperative CT is acquired to further define the anatomy of the intrahepatic biliary tree and the distal common bile duct [13]. MR cholangiography may also be useful in the preoperative anatomic assessment of these lesions [10–12].

Spontaneous perforation of the extrahepatic bile ducts

Spontaneous perforation of the extrahepatic bile ducts is a cause of neonatal jaundice and ascites, usually affecting infants between 1 week and 4 months of age. The clinical findings include ascites, mild jaundice, failure to thrive, and abdominal distension. The serum bilirubin level is elevated, whereas other liver function tests are normal. The latter feature is helpful in differentiating perforation from neonatal hepatitis and biliary atresia, which have similar clinical findings but abnormal liver function tests. The most frequent site of perforation is the junction of the cystic and common bile ducts. Rarely the perforation involves the common hepatic duct, gallbladder, or junction of the cystic duct and gallbladder [30].

Sonography shows generalized ascites or a loculated fluid collection in the porta hepatis [30] (**Fig. 7**). Echogenic debris or fine septations may be present within the ascitic fluid. The biliary tree is not dilated because it is not obstructed. Gallbladder or distal common duct calculi may be associated findings. Hepatobiliary scintigraphy is useful to confirm the diagnosis by showing leaking of radioactive tracer into the peritoneal cavity. Surgical

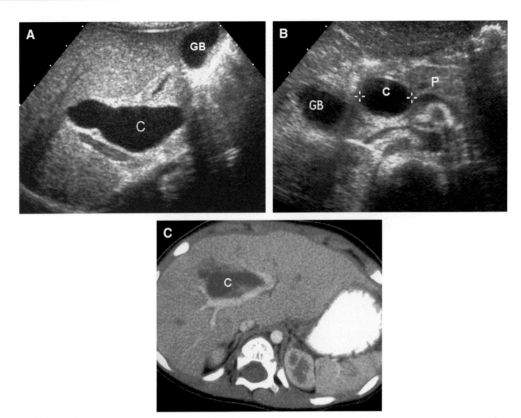

Fig. 6. Choledochal cyst in a young boy with jaundice. (*A*) Longitudinal and (*B*) transverse sonograms through the liver demonstrate a cystic mass (C), representing the choledochal cyst, in the porta hepatis separate from the gallbladder (GB). P, pancreas. (*C*) Contrast-enhanced CT scan confirms the cystic mass (C), which is the dilated common bile duct.

placement of a drainage tube in the area of perforation usually results in spontaneous closure.

Inspissated bile syndrome

The inspissated bile or bile-plug syndrome refers to an extrahepatic obstruction of the bile ducts by biliary sludge [2]. This condition typically affects full-term infants. Inspissated bile syndrome has been associated with massive hemolysis, hemorrhage, total parenteral nutrition, cystic fibrosis, and various intestinal diseases (Hirschsprung disease, intestinal atresias, and stenoses). Sonography shows moderately or highly echogenic bile within the gallbladder and often within dilated intra- or extrahepatic bile ducts. Although the bile is echogenic, it does not cause acoustic shadowing. The ductal dilatation may be difficult to recognize if the echogenicity of the inspissated bile and liver are similar [1,2].

Jaundice in older infants and children

The causes of jaundice in older children and adolescents include cystic diseases, including choledochal cyst (see earlier discussion) and Caroli disease, diseases of the hepatocytes, and inflammatory and obstructive lesions of the biliary ducts.

Caroli disease

Caroli disease, also known as congenital cystic dilation of the intrahepatic biliary tract, has two forms. One form is characterized by segmental, saccular dilation of the intrahepatic bile ducts, an increased frequency of calculus formation and cholangitis, and the absence of cirrhosis and portal hypertension. The other form is characterized by hepatic fibrosis, cirrhosis, and portal hypertension. Both forms of Caroli disease are associated with renal cystic disease, including renal tubular ectasia (medullary sponge kidney), cortical cysts, and autosomal recessive polycystic disease. Patients who have Caroli disease, like those who have choledochal cysts, have an increased risk for developing cholangiocarcinoma. Patients may present in the neonatal period [31], but the vast majority present as young adults who have abdominal pain, fever, and jaundice or with portal hypertension.

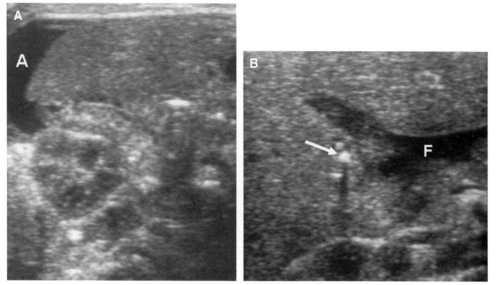

Fig. 7. Spontaneous perforation of the common bile duct. (*A*) Transverse sonogram through the upper abdomen demonstrates ascites (A) in the perihepatic space. (*B*) On a more caudad image, a loculated fluid (F) collection and a calculus (*arrow*) are noted in the porta hepatis.

Sonography shows multiple dilated tubular structures, typical of biliary radicals (Fig. 8). These can converge, creating larger saccular areas [31]. The portal radicals may be partially or completely surrounded by the dilated ducts (termed the central dot sign) [32] (Fig. 9). The extrahepatic bile ducts can be normal, narrowed, or associated with a choledochal cyst. Findings of portal hypertension may be observed in patients who have hepatic fibrosis.

Byler disease

Byler syndrome (also known as progressive familial intrahepatic fibrosis) is a familial intrahepatic cholestatic syndrome that is associated with cystic hepatic lesions and jaundice. Histologically, there is periportal fibrosis, micronodular cirrhosis, and periductal cysts. Symptoms, including jaundice, pruritus, and hepatomegaly, usually appear by the end of the first year of life. The sonographic findings

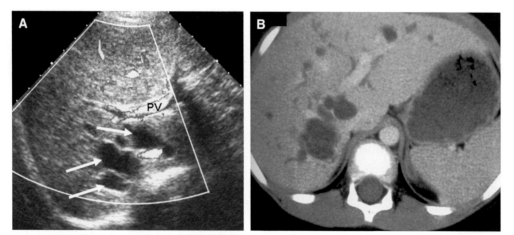

Fig. 8. Caroli disease. (*A*) Transverse Doppler sonogram shows dilatation of the intrahepatic bile ducts (*arrows*), which converge toward the porta hepatis. The color Doppler image helps confirm the absence of flow in the dilated ducts. Flow is seen in the portal vein (PV). (*B*) CT confirms saccular dilatation of the bile ducts. (*From* Siegel MJ. Gallbladder and biliary tract. In: Siegel MJ, editor. Pediatric sonography. 3rd edition. Philadelphia: Lippincott Williams & Wilkins; 2002. p. 276–304; with permission).

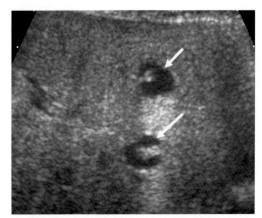

Fig. 9. Caroli disease. Transverse sonogram shows dilated ducts (*arrows*) that completely envelope the portal radicals. This appearance is termed the central dot sign.

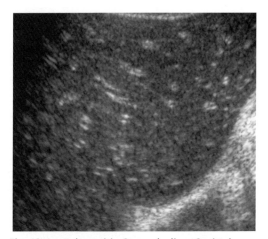

Fig. 10. Acute hepatitis. Starry sky liver. Sagittal sonogram of the liver shows brightly echogenic portal venous triads. The liver was also moderately enlarged.

are multiple saccular cystic lesions, some of which may contain echogenic portal veins (the central dot sign) [33]. Unlike Caroli disease, the cysts in Byler disease do not communicate with the bile ducts.

Hepatocellular diseases

Hepatocellular disease can be classified into two major classes: infectious (acute and chronic hepatitis) and noninfectious (metabolic disorders, drugs, toxins, and autoimmune diseases). The sonographic appearance of the liver depends on the severity of the insult, rather than on the causative agent [1]. Sonography is usually normal in cases of mild acute infectious hepatitis. Sonographic findings in severe acute hepatitis include hepatomegaly, decreased parenchymal echogenicity, and increased echogenicity of the portal venule walls (starry sky liver) (Fig. 10). The gallbladder wall may be small, thick-walled, and filled with intraluminal sludge. In chronic active hepatitis, the liver often appears heterogeneous and hyperechoic with irregular margins and decreased visualization of the portal venous radicles (Fig. 11). The gallbladder may be small and contain thick bile, sludge, or stones, and collateral vessel formation may be noted.

Metabolic causes of jaundice include Wilson disease, cystic fibrosis, glycogen storage disease, tyrosinemia, and α_1-antitrypsin deficiency. The sonographic appearance of these disorders is nonspecific and can be similar to that of acute or chronic hepatitis. A definitive diagnosis requires correlation with clinical information and laboratory results, and in many cases biopsy is needed to confirm the diagnosis.

Inflammatory diseases of the biliary ducts

Sclerosing cholangitis

Sclerosing cholangitis is a chronic cholestatic disorder characterized by inflammatory obliterative fibrosis of the extrahepatic and intrahepatic bile ducts leading to biliary cirrhosis and ultimately liver failure [34]. This entity has been associated with chronic inflammatory bowel disease, Langerhans histiocytosis X, and immunodeficiency disorders [34]. Histologic examination shows multiple segmental strictures, diverticula formation between areas of stricture, and mural thickening of the bile ducts. Clinical manifestations include jaundice and right upper quadrant pain. Most affected patients are adolescents or adults.

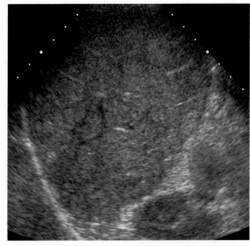

Fig. 11. Chronic hepatitis. Longitudinal sonogram of the liver shows an enlarged liver with irregular margins and diffusely coarse echotexture.

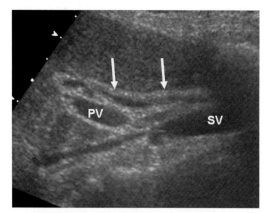

Fig. 12. Sclerosing cholangitis. Longitudinal sonogram shows a dilated, thick-walled common bile duct (*arrows*) (diameter, 9 mm). PV, portal vein; SV, splenic vein.

Sonographic findings include a thick-walled gallbladder, thick-walled dilated intrahepatic ducts (Fig. 12), intrahepatic and intraductal stones, cholelithiasis, and segmental ductal narrowing secondary to stricturing. The strictures may be difficult to detect sonographically unless the ducts are dilated. In longstanding disease, sonography may show findings of biliary cirrhosis and portal hypertension.

AIDS-related cholangitis

The common biliary tract abnormalities in children who have AIDS are acalculous cholecystitis and cholangitis. The sonographic findings in AIDS-related cholangitis are similar to those of sclerosing cholangitis and include ductal dilatation and wall irregularity (Fig. 13), stricture of the intra- and extrahepatic bile ducts, and a dilated, thick-walled gallbladder wall [35–37]. An additional finding is a hyperechoic nodule in the distal end of the common bile duct caused by edema of the papilla of Vater [38].

Biliary tract obstruction

Sonographic features

Biliary obstruction resulting in jaundice is usually the result of stone disease. Acute pancreatitis, neoplasm, and benign strictures are less common causes of obstructive jaundice in children. The sonographic diagnosis of biliary obstruction is based on the demonstration of dilated intrahepatic or extrahepatic bile ducts. Dilated intrahepatic biliary radicles appear as multiple, anechoic branching structures that enlarge as they approach the porta hepatis. The dilated common hepatic and common bile ducts may appear as round or tubular anechoic structures near the porta hepatis or the head of the pancreas (Fig. 13).

Cholelithiasis and choledocholithiasis

Stones in the common bile duct usually originate in the gallbladder and migrate distally. Cholelithiasis in neonates has been associated with congenital anomalies of the biliary tract, total parenteral nutrition, furosemide therapy, phototherapy, dehydration, infection, hemolytic anemias, and short-gut syndrome [9]. In older children, causes of cholelithiasis include sickle cell disease, cystic fibrosis, malabsorption, total parenteral nutrition, liver disease, Crohn disease, bowel resection, and hemolytic anemia.

Choledocholithiasis typically manifests as brightly echogenic shadowing foci within the

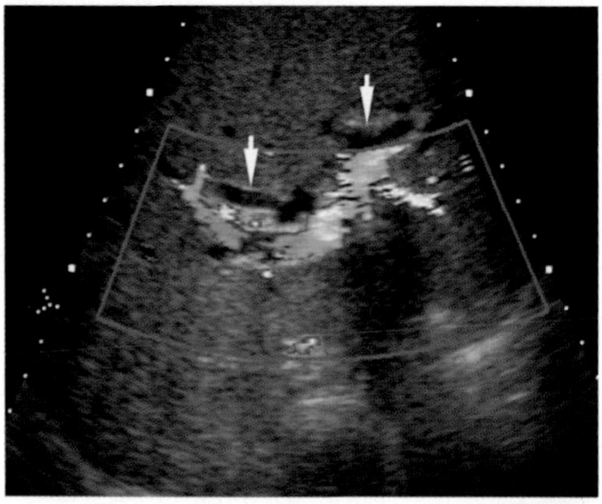

Fig. 13. AIDS-related cholangitis. Longitudinal sonogram at the level of the porta hepatitis demonstrates intrahepatic ductal dilatation (*arrows*). (Courtesy of Edward Lee, MD, Boston, MA).

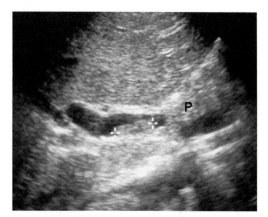

Fig. 14. Choledocholithiasis. Longitudinal scan at the level of the pancreatic head (P) shows a stone (*between calipers*) without shadowing. At operation, calcium bilirubinate stones were found in the gallbladder and distal duct. Ductal diameter is 11 mm.

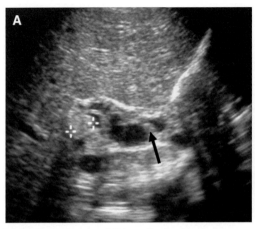 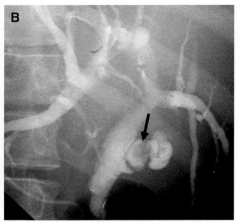

Fig. 15. Cystic duct stone. (*A*) Longitudinal scan shows a calculus (*calipers*) in the cystic duct. A second calculus (*arrow*) is noted in the distal common bile duct, which is dilated. (*B*) Endoscopic retrograde cholangiogram confirms the stone (*arrow*) in the cystic duct. (*From* Siegel MJ. Gallbladder and biliary tract. In: Siegel MJ, editor. Pediatric sonography. 3rd edition. Philadelphia: Lippincott Williams & Wilkins; 2002. p. 276–304; with permission).

biliary ducts and is usually associated with ductal dilatation (Fig. 14). The calculi obstruct anywhere in the biliary duct, but most cause obstruction at the level of the pancreatic head. The sensitivity for detection of choledocholithiasis is lower for stones in the distal versus the proximal duct. A calculus impacted in the distal duct can be more difficult to detect because of adjacent or overlying bowel gas and because the calculus is surrounded by the echogenic pancreatic head.

Cystic duct stones
Mirizzi syndrome is a rare cause of biliary obstruction in children. It is secondary to an impacted cystic duct stone, which causes extrinsic compression or inflammatory stricture of the common duct. Sonographic findings include calculi in the gallbladder neck or in the cystic duct and dilated intrahepatic ducts, including the common hepatic duct (Fig. 15).

Biliary neoplasms
Rhabdomyosarcoma of the biliary tract is rare, but it is the most common neoplasm of the biliary tract in children. Most rhabdomyosarcomas arise in the porta hepatis and involve the cystic duct. Sonographic findings are intra- and extrahepatic ductal dilatation and an echogenic mass without acoustic shadowing. Rhabdomyosarcoma spreads by direct extension to contiguous structures or by hematogenous or lymphatic dissemination to lymph nodes, lungs, bone, bone marrow, or liver.

Biliary duct strictures
Biliary stricture is an uncommon cause of distal obstruction, but the diagnosis needs to be considered in patients who have biliary obstruction in whom no calculus or other obstructing lesion can be visualized. An abrupt transition from a dilated duct to one of normal caliber is a finding suggestive of stricture.

References

[1] Gubernick JA, Rosenberg HK, Ilaslan H, et al. US approach to jaundice in infants and children. Radiographics 2000;20:173–95.
[2] Siegel MJ. Gallbladder and biliary tract. In: Siegel MJ, editor. Pediatric sonography. 3rd edition. Philadelphia: Lippincott Williams & Wilkins; 2002. p. 276–304.
[3] Hernanz-Schulman M, Ambrosino MM, Freeman PC, et al. Common bile duct in children: sonographic dimensions. Radiology 1982; 145:437.
[4] Wachsberg RH. Respiratory variation of extrahepatic bile duct diameter during ultrasonography. J Ultrasound Med 1994;13:617.
[5] Wolson AH. Ultrasound measurements of the gallbladder. In: Goldberg BB, Kurtz AB, editors. Atlas of ultrasound measurements. Chicago: Year Book Publishers, Inc.; 1990. p. 108–12.
[6] Siegel MJ, Martin KW, Worthington JL. Normal and abnormal pancreas in children: US studies. Radiology 1987;165:15–8.
[7] Balistreri WF, Grand R, Hoofnagle JH, et al. Biliary atresia: current concepts and research directions. Summary of a symposium. Hepatology 1996;23:1682–90.
[8] Balistreri WF, Schubert WK. Liver diseases in infancy and childhood. In: Schiff L, Schiff ER, editors. Diseases of the liver. 7th edition. Philadelphia: JB Lippincott; 1993. p. 1099–203.

[9] Roberts EA. The jaundiced baby. In: Kelly DA, editor. Diseases of the liver and biliary system in children. Oxford UK: Blackwell Science; 1999. p. 11–45.

[10] Guibaud L, Lachaud A, Touraine R, et al. MR cholangiography in neonates and infants: feasibility and preliminary applications. Am J Roentgenol 1998;170:27–31.

[11] Irie H, Honda H, Jimi M, et al. Value of MR cholangiopancreatography in evaluating choledochal cysts. Am J Roentgenol 1998;171:1381–5.

[12] Miyazaki T, Yamashita Y, Tang Y, et al. Single-shot MR cholangiopancreatography of neonates, infants, and young children. Am J Roentgenol 1998; 170:33–7.

[13] Siegel MJ. Liver and biliary tract. In: Siegel MJ, editor. Pediatric body CT. Philadelphia: Lippincott Williams Wilkins; 1999. p. 141–74.

[14] Siegel MJ. Pediatric liver imaging. Semin Liver Dis 2001;21:251–69.

[15] Roy CC, Silverman A, Alagille D. Pediatric clinical gastroenterology. St. Louis: Mosby; 1995.

[16] Abramson SJ, Berdon WE, Altman RP, et al. Biliary atresia and noncardiac polysplenic syndrome: US and surgical considerations. Radiology 1987; 163:377–9.

[17] Kim WS, Kim IO, Yeon KM, et al. Choledochal cyst with or without biliary atresia in neonates and young infants: US differentiation. Radiology 1998;209:465–9.

[18] Torrisi JM, Haller JO, Velcek FT. Choledochal cyst and biliary atresia in the neonate: imaging findings in five cases. Am J Roentgenol 1990; 155:1273–6.

[19] Carceller A, Blanchard H, Alvarez F, et al. Past and future of biliary atresia. J Pediatr Surg 2000;35:717–20.

[20] Choi S-O, Park W-H, Lee H-J, et al. "Triangular cord": a sonographic finding applicable in the diagnosis of biliary atresia. J Pediatr Surg 1996; 31:363–6.

[21] Kendrick APT, Phua KB, Subramaniam R, et al. Making the diagnosis of biliary atresia using the triangular cord sign and gallbladder length. Pediatr Radiol 2000;30:69–73.

[22] Park W-H, Choi S-O, Lee H-J, et al. A new diagnostic approach to biliary atresia with emphasis on the ultrasonographic triangular cord sign: comparison of ultrasonography, hepatobiliary scintigraphy, and liver needle biopsy in the evaluation of infantile cholestasis. J Pediatr Surg 1997;32:1555–9.

[23] Park W-H, Choi S-O, Lee H-J. The ultrasonographic "triangular cord" couples with gallbladder images in the diagnostic prediction of biliary atresia from infantile intrahepatic cholestasis. J Pedatr Surg 1999;34:1706–10.

[24] Ikeda S, Sera Y, Ohshiro H, et al. Gallbladder contraction in biliary atresia: a pitfall of ultrasound diagnosis. Pediatr Radiol 1998;28:451–3.

[25] Weinberger E, Blumhagen JD, Odell JM. Gallbladder contraction in biliary atresia. Am J Roentgenol 1987;149:401–2.

[26] Alagille D, Estrada A, Hadchouel M, et al. Syndromic paucity of interlobular bile ducts (Alagille syndrome or arteriohepatic dysplasia): review of 80 cases. J Pediatr 1987;110: 195–200.

[27] Kim OH, Chung HJ, Choi BG. Imaging of the choledochal cyst. Radiographics 1995;15:69–88.

[28] Babbitt DP, Starshak RJ, Clemett AR. Choledochal cyst: a concept of etiology. Am J Roentgenol 1973;119:57–62.

[29] Savader SJ, Benenati JF, Venbrux AC, et al. Choledochal cysts: classification and cholangiographic appearance. Am J Roentgenol 1991; 156:327–31.

[30] Haller JO, Conden VR, Berdon WE, et al. Spontaneous perforation of the common bile duct in children. Radiology 1989;172:621–4.

[31] Toma P, Lucigrai G, Pelizza A. Sonographic patterns of Caroli's disease: report of 5 new cases. J Clin Ultrasound 1991;19:155–61.

[32] Miller WJ, Sechtin AG, Campbell WL, et al. Imaging findings in Caroli's disease. Am J Roentgenol 1995;165:333–7.

[33] Herman TE, Siegel MJ. Central dot sign on CT of liver cysts. J Comput Assist Tomogr 1990; 14:1019–21.

[34] Debray D, Pariente D, Urvoas E, et al. Sclerosing cholangitis in children. J Pediatr 1994;124: 49–56.

[35] Chung CJ, Sivit CJ, Rakusan TA, et al. Hepatobiliary abnormalities on sonography in children with HIV infection. J Ultrasound Med 1994; 13:205–10.

[36] Dolmatch BL, Laing FC, Federle MP, et al. AIDS-related cholangitis: radiographic findings in nine patients. Radiology 1987;163:313.

[37] Grumbach K, Coleman BG, Gal AA, et al. Hepatic and biliary tract abnormalities in patients with AIDS. Sonographic-pathologic correlation. J Ultrasound Med 1989;8:247–54.

[38] Da Silva F, Boudghene F, Lecomte I, et al. Sonography in AIDS-related cholangitis: prevalence and cause of an echogenic nodule in the distal end of the common bile duct. Am J Roentgenol 1993;160:1205–7.

ELSEVIER
SAUNDERS

ULTRASOUND
CLINICS

Ultrasound Clin 1 (2006) 443–455

Pediatric Portal Hypertension

Zoltan Harkanyi, MD, PhD

The incidence of portal hypertension (PHT) in the pediatric age group has fortunately decreased in the past decades, in contrast to adults, for whom the number of affected patients has dramatically increased. This phenomenon is a sign of improved neonatal care and earlier diagnosis of conditions leading to PHT.

Despite progress in the treatment of variceal bleeding and other complications related to PHT, elevated portal pressure still represents a great danger to affected pediatric patients. The mortality associated with bleeding is still approximately 20% at 6 weeks [1].

PHT is defined as a pathologic increase of portal venous pressure that can be characterized by the hepatic vein pressure gradient. If the value of the pressure gradient is greater than 5 mm Hg, PHT is present. This measurement is still the best predictor of the development of varices and ascites [1,2]. Unfortunately no imaging modality is able to measure actual portal venous pressure, and invasive techniques are required for direct measurements in the portal and hepatic veins or in the inferior vena cava.

The role of conventional two-dimensional (2D) and Doppler ultrasound (US) in the evaluation of PHT has been extensively studied in the past 25 years and its significance can be summarized as follows:

(1) US can evaluate the whole abdomen, including the size of the liver and spleen, any parenchymal abnormalities, and the presence of any free abdominal fluid.
(2) US shows the anatomy of the portal venous system, the hepatic veins, the hepatic artery (HA), and the inferior vena cava.
(3) US provides clinically relevant functional information on the actual hemodynamic status of the patient. All observations and measurements can be done with an unlimited time window compared with CT or MR

Department of Radiology, Heim Pal Children's Hospital, 1089 Budapest, Ulloi ut 86, Hungary
E-mail address: zoharkanyi@yahoo.com

1556-858X/06/$ – see front matter © 2006 Elsevier Inc. All rights reserved.
ultrasound.theclinics.com

doi:10.1016/j.cult.2006.05.003

imaging. US causes no harm to the patient (radiation, IV contrast agents) and is available worldwide.

Applications of imaging in PHT include:

(1) Establishing or supporting the clinical diagnosis of PHT. Patients who have a known risk for developing PHT (eg, portal vein occlusion, diffuse liver disease) should be scanned on a regular basis. Rarely, US can detect signs of PHT incidentally during an abdominal or pelvic study (pelvic varices).

(2) Selecting cases before, during, and after various treatments (sclerotherapy, transjugular intrahepatic portosystemic shunt [TIPS], surgical shunt procedures).

(3) Following patients who have known PHT to demonstrate portosystemic collaterals and the flow direction and patency of the splenoportal veins.

Ultrasound imaging in portal hypertension

In the past decades, US imaging has played a leading role in the evaluation of patients who have known or suspected PHT, because liver disease, hepatic vessels, and hemodynamics should be studied at the same time. High-resolution 2D imaging, color Doppler imaging, and duplex Doppler has been used (Table 1).

Power Doppler, 3D/4D US, and B-flow imaging are useful additional newer tools, though the application of these options is not an essential part of the evaluation. US contrast studies have shown promising preliminary results in adult patients who have cirrhosis, PHT, and portal vein thrombosis. US contrast agents, however, remain currently unavailable and unapproved for use in the pediatric age group.

Two-dimensional ultrasonography

It is a logical approach to start an examination with a detailed 2D imaging of the abdomen in all cases. Tissue harmonic imaging has become a routine option on almost all US systems and should also be used whenever needed in pediatric patients. High-resolution convex or sector probes are typically used. Linear transducers can give additional information regarding the liver surface in parenchymal disorders and can also demonstrate superficial varices in the abdominal wall (caput medusae).

The size, shape, and echotexture of the liver and the spleen should be studied and documented. Two-dimensional gray-scale imaging often reveals the presence of collaterals, the size and anatomy of the splenoportal veins, and shows ascites in advanced cases. Real-time scanning allows observation of the respiratory changes of the size of the portal vein, superior mesenteric vein (SMV), and the inferior vena cava (IVC).

Color Doppler imaging and duplex Doppler

All three hepatic vascular systems should be studied to search for the signs of PHT (Fig. 1). The scan parameters must be adjusted to the patient's body habitus and the types of the vessels under study. In PHT, very slow flow can be present in the portal vein, thus pulse repetition frequency (PRF), velocity, scale, wall filter, and Doppler gain should be modified according to the actual flow condition. The flow sensitivity of new color Doppler systems has improved dramatically. The presence and the direction of flow are easily seen with good temporal and spatial resolution, and motion artifacts have diminished.

Duplex Doppler is usually applied at selected vessel segments to document the direction, type, and velocity of flow. Sometimes it is difficult or even impossible to obtain sufficient Doppler waveforms during breathholding in small babies and young children. In these cases one may have to rely on the color Doppler findings. New color systems allow continuous observation during respiration.

The main portal vein and the major lobar branches must be examined and documented. Intercostal scanning is often necessary to visualize the vessels and flow direction properly. The normal main portal vein should be seen in 100% of cases.

Table 1: Ultrasound imaging in portal hypertension	
Ultrasound method	**Function**
2D US imaging	Basic method: vessel anatomy, liver/spleen parenchyma
Color Doppler imaging (CDI), Power Doppler imaging (PDI)	Patency of the veins, direction and type of flow
Duplex Doppler	Doppler waveform analysis, Flow velocity measurements, Calculated flow parameters (VPI, RI)
3D/4D US and multiplanar US imaging	3D display of the hepatic vessel anatomy and vascular anomalies
Endoscopic/endoluminal US	Detection of gastroesophageal varices

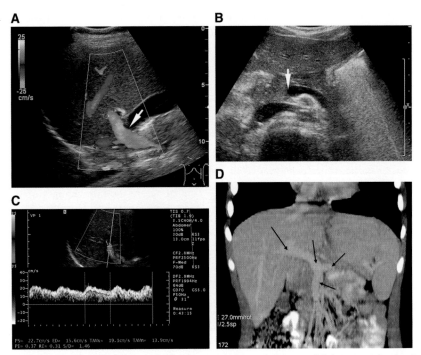

Fig. 1. Ultrasound demonstration of the normal splenoportal venous system. (*A*) Intercostal color Doppler sonogram shows a normal main portal vein (*arrow*). (*B*) Mesenterico-splenic junction (*arrow*), transverse image. (*C*) Duplex image of the main portal vein. The Doppler spectrum is recorded during breathhold. Using Doppler shift measurement with angle correction, the actual flow velocity and venous pulsatility index (VPI) can be calculated. (*D*) The sites of Doppler sampling are indicated (*arrows*) on a coronal reconstructed CT image.

Doppler waveform analysis and angle-corrected velocity determination should be performed.

The splenic vein is best seen in the hilum of the spleen. The superior mesenteric vein is sometimes hidden by overlying bowel gas; however, the confluence of the SMV and the splenic vein is usually visualized posterior to the pancreas. Gentle mechanical compression of the bowel can be helpful to find an acoustic window to visualize the SMV and splenic vein.

The left, right, and middle hepatic veins should be examined and followed to the IVC. A good temporal resolution color Doppler system should reveal normal triphasic flow. A biphasic or monophasic hepatic vein waveform can indicate parenchymal liver disease (see later discussion) (Fig. 2). Anatomic variation of the hepatic veins is frequent, and in 25% to 30% of the cases more than three hepatic veins are present.

Evaluation of IVC is also part of the standard Doppler study. The vessel usually is well visualized running from the right atrium inferiorly, posterior to the liver.

Generally the HA can be well visualized in the porta hepatis. Although the flow direction is the same in the HA and in the portal vein, a clear distinction can be made using a high-resolution US system. Doppler waveform analysis is also part of the hepatic study and resistance index (RI) measurements can be performed.

Other ultrasound techniques

Power Doppler imaging was originally suggested for the detection of slow flow in small caliber vessels, and some newer US systems are even able to show flow direction using power Doppler. Using a high-sensitivity conventional color Doppler system, all three hepatic vascular systems can be evaluated. Power Doppler imaging is generally not needed, because no additional information is obtained.

B-flow imaging is a new approach in the demonstration of flow in abdominal vessels, including the portal system. No definitive advantage of this method has been proven so far.

The technology of 3D/4D and multiplanar ultrasound has significantly improved in the past years. Volume US acquisition of a given organ and especially 3D real-time observation of the vasculature may be helpful in understanding complex intrahepatic vascular anatomy in selected cases [3]. Real time 3D US technology is still a work in progress, but the quality of the reconstructed images will no doubt be further improved.

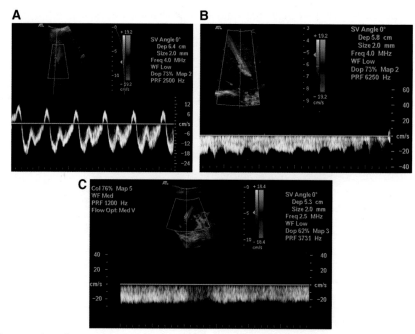

Fig. 2. Duplex Doppler of normal and abnormal hepatic veins. (*A*) Normal triphasic hepatic vein waveform in a healthy child. (*B*) Biphasic Doppler waveform, which can be a sign of parenchymal liver disease. (*C*) Monophasic Doppler spectrum.

Ultrasound contrast agents in conjunction with special software (contrast harmonic imaging) can be used to measure hepatic transit time and to detect portal vein thrombosis in adults [4]. The reported results are promising in hepatic cirrhosis, but the technique has not yet achieved routine clinical use. Routine US contrast use in pediatric patients awaits further testing.

Endoscopic and endoluminal US using high frequency special probes are accurate in demonstrating gastroesophageal (GE) varices. Collaterals not seen during endoscopy because of their deeper position can be detected with US. The pediatric application of this technique is limited because of patient size and the need for sedation.

Causes and types of portal hypertension

The well-known classification of PHT is also valid for the pediatric age group: prehepatic, hepatic, and posthepatic (Table 2). In the vast majority of pediatric patients, prehepatic causes occur because of occlusion of splenoportal veins for various reasons. Congenital hepatic fibrosis is the second leading cause, and less frequently other diffuse parenchymal liver diseases can cause elevated portal

Table 2: Types and causes of portal hypertension in pediatric patients

Prehepatic	Inflow obstruction	Portal vein, mesenteric vein thrombosis
		Portal vein compression
Intrahepatic	Increased intrahepatic resistance	Diffuse parenchymal liver disease (hepatic fibrosis, cirrhosis)
		Liver tumors
Posthepatic	Outflow obstruction	Hepatic vein thrombosis (Budd-Chiari syndrome)
		IVC web
		Hepatic veno-occlusive disease
		Congestive heart failure

pressure. The posthepatic causes are rare in childhood.

Portal vein thrombosis—prehepatic portal hypertension

There are three main etiologic factors of portal vein obstruction: infection, hypercoagulable state, and tumor invasion [5,6].

(1) Neonatal umbilical infection is mainly related to umbilical vein catheterization, but it can occur without external intervention. Portal thrombosis also occurs after complicated acute appendicitis, long-standing inflammatory bowel disease (especially Crohn disease), or other abdominal and pelvic inflammatory processes.

(2) Hematologic disorders, such as protein C, protein S, antithrombin III, or factor V Leyden deficiency may present with thromboses. Hypercoagulable states can occur with sepsis, dehydration, and nephrotic syndrome.

(3) Though primary liver tumors are rare conditions in children, direct vessel invasion and compression can occur in cases of hepatoblastoma or hepatocellular carcinoma.

Several studies support the suspicion that there is a strong connection between neonatal umbilical vein catheterization and development of portal vein thrombosis. In one study, US revealed portal vein thrombus in 43% of catheterized neonates [7]. Low birth weight and long-standing umbilical catheterization increase the risk for thrombus development, which can be monitored with US.

Portal vein thrombosis is usually easily recognized with US as an echogenic solid mass within an enlarged portal vein. In such cases color Doppler reveals a complete absence of flow. In partial portal vein thrombosis, very slow flow is present in the affected vessel segment (Fig. 3). When the thrombus is fresh and hypoechoic, it poses a potential pitfall of US diagnosis of PHT. In chronic cases, the echogenicity of the thrombus can be equivalent to the surrounding liver parenchyma. In doubtful cases, contrast-enhanced CT or MR imaging can solve the diagnostic problem.

The most typical form of chronic portal vein thrombosis in childhood is the development of cavernous transformation of the portal vein, when numerous small collaterals develop in the porta hepatis and sometimes within the liver parenchyma (Fig. 4). The portal cavernoma is usually well visualized on 2D US, and color Doppler proves the presence of slow venous flow in these tiny vessels. The enlarged HA should be differentiated from the venous collaterals. The normal main portal vein and the right portal vein must be seen in all patients, even uncooperative infants and children. If the detection of flow in these portal branches is not possible, the suspicion of portal vein occlusion should be raised. Again, contrast-enhanced CT and MR imaging may be helpful in questionable cases. Patients who have portal cavernoma rarely develop other portosystemic collaterals, implying that the venous circulation can adapt to this condition.

Diffuse parenchymal liver disease—intrahepatic portal hypertension

Long-standing increased intrahepatic resistance gradually leads to PHT and development of portosystemic collaterals. Increased intrahepatic vascular resistance can be the cause of PHT in congenital hepatic fibrosis, cystic fibrosis, autosomal recessive polycystic renal disease associated with fibrosis, biliary atresia, and primary sclerosing cholangitis. Untreated or undetected biliary atresia can also lead to fibrosis; the US morphology is similar to congenital liver fibrosis. In contrast to adults, cirrhosis, chronic hepatitis, and infectious hepatitis are rare causes of PHT in children.

Sonography is unfortunately not specific enough to detect early signs of parenchymal liver disease, and differentiation between fatty liver changes

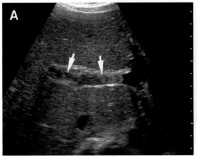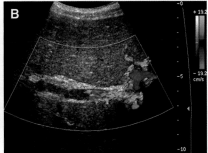

Fig. 3. Portal vein thrombosis. (*A*) Echogenic mass (*arrows*) represents chronic thrombus in the right portal vein. (*B*) Color Doppler proves complete occlusion of the vessel.

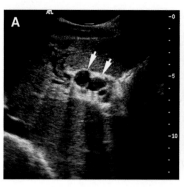
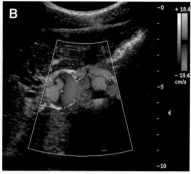

Fig. 4. Portal cavernoma, portal vein thrombosis. (A) Multiple cystic structures (*arrows*) are seen in the porta hepatis on this subcostal US gray-scale image. Cavernous transformation of the portal vein is generally a consequence of complete occlusion of the main portal vein. (B) Color Doppler demonstrates slow venous flow in the collaterals.

and hepatic fibrosis is especially difficult using ultrasound.

In advanced cases of parenchymal liver disease, the US appearance is typical: increased echogenicity; coarse, heterogeneous echotexture; irregular liver surface (best seen using a linear transducer); compression of the thin-walled hepatic veins; and narrowing of the portal vein branches. The spleen can be enlarged, and with severe disease ascites is present. The size and shape of the liver should be analyzed carefully. The enlargement of segment 1 (caudate lobe) because of its special hemodynamics can be a sensitive indicator of diffuse liver disease. In advanced disease the right lobe is small.

Intrahepatic vascular malformations can have hemodynamic effects on portal venous and hepatic arterial circulation, which can be evaluated by duplex Doppler. Portosystemic shunts and arterioportal shunts can be found with gray-scale and color Doppler, and in some cases pose a risk for development of PHT (Fig. 5) [8].

Outflow obstruction—posthepatic portal hypertension

Outflow obstruction is a rare cause of PHT in children, usually caused by underlying thrombosis. Hepatic vein thrombosis (Budd-Chiari syndrome) has characteristic US signs: echogenic material in the hepatic vein and no flow visible using color Doppler (Fig. 6). Enlargement of the caudate lobe (segment 1) is a typical finding. An inferior vena cava

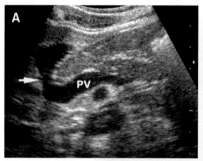
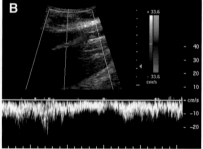
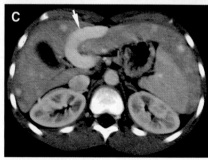

Fig. 5. Persistent ductus venosus. Persistent ductus venosus represents a congenital communication between the portal vein and the systemic circulation. (A) Transverse US image shows the dilated left portal vein (PV) and the persistent ductus venosus (*arrow*) entering into the IVC. (B) Duplex Doppler shows continuous flow within the vessel. (C) Contrast-enhanced CT image shows the dilated left portal vein (*arrow*).

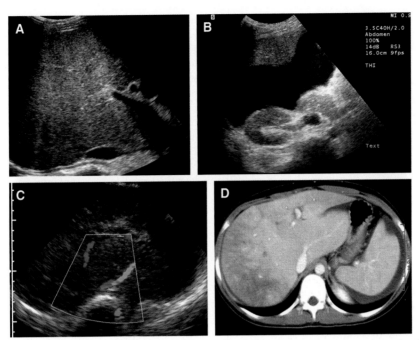

Fig. 6. Hepatic vein thrombosis. (*A*) Subcostal 2D images in a patient who had sudden onset of ascites show inhomogeneous liver parenchyma, and (*B*) ascites. (*C*) Color Doppler shows flow in the left and middle hepatic veins, but no flow in the right hepatic vein. (*D*) The corresponding contrast-enhanced CT confirmed the findings of right hepatic vein thrombosis. The echogenicity (US) and the density (CT) are different in the two lobes of the liver. In this patient who had Budd-Chiari syndrome, portal hypertension developed gradually.

membrane (or hepatic web) is a rare cause of venous outflow or postsinusoidal obstruction.

Hepatic veno-occlusive disease is mainly related to bone marrow transplantation in the pediatric age. The disorder causes progressive occlusion of the small hepatic venules, and the clinical presentation is similar to Budd-Chiari syndrome. Sonography can show abnormal portal flow, which may be hepatofugal or biphasic in the main portal vein. Hepatic vein and IVC flow may be preserved [9].

Qualitative ultrasound evaluation of portal hypertension

It would be desirable to measure the actual portal venous pressure with sonography. Unfortunately, US is able to measure the vessel size and flow velocity only, and with limited accuracy the portal flow volume can be determined using various Doppler methods.

The US signs of portal hypertension are summarized in Box 1.

The hemodynamic changes induced by elevated portal pressure are a complicated process during the progress of the underlying disease, and no single US measurement provides a reliable parameter for establishing the diagnosis. The actual measurement of portal flow is also influenced by various factors. The respiratory phase of the measurement, cardiac output, tricuspid regurgitation, eating–fasting, and position of the patient, among other factors, influence the results. Portal flow velocity decreases during the progression of PHT, and flow volume is highly dependent on the number and size of diverting portosystemic collaterals. Increasing arterial inflow by way of the HA gradually compensates

---

Box 1: Vascular ultrasound signs of portal hypertension

- Porto-systemic collaterals
- Hepatofugal flow/bidirectional flow
- Decreased portal flow velocity
- Decreased portal flow volume
- Decreased pulsatility of portal flow (VPI)
- Dilatation of the central portal vessels, narrowing of the peripheral branches
- No increase of portal flow velocity and volume after meal
- Compression of the hepatic veins: 'pseudoportal flow'
- Enlargement and tortuosity of the hepatic artery
- Hepatic artery: increased RI, increased flow volume
- Arterio-portal shunting

for the decrease in portal blood flow. Arterial flow volume and HA resistance typically increase as part of the hemodynamic changes.

Portosystemic collaterals: key findings in portal hypertension

The qualitative evaluation of the portal circulation probably has the greatest clinical significance. One of the most important goals of the US examination in PHT is to detect the presence of portosystemic collaterals in different localizations (Fig. 7). This is the most sensitive (70%–83%) and specific (100%) sonographic finding in PHT [2,10].

The most obvious sites of the collaterals are the gastroesophageal varices, the left coronary vein, splenorenal shunts, and the recanalized paraumbilical vein. The degree of PHT correlates with the number of shunts [10,11] (Fig. 8).

If dilated, the left gastric vein (coronary vein) can be well visualized posterior to the left lobe of the liver (Fig. 8A); it is an important finding because it is related to the development of esophageal varices [11,12]. Color Doppler is more sensitive and accurate in the depiction of the collaterals than gray-scale US. With proper examination technique, collaterals can be observed in the retroperitoneum,

in the gall bladder wall (which may be thickened with PHT), and in the pelvis. The location and the size of the portosystemic collaterals have prognostic importance in cirrhotics; patients who have large shunts toward the inferior vena cava have fewer or no esophageal varices [13].

The paraumbilical vein in the falciform ligament connects the intrahepatic portal branches with the inferior epigastric veins of the abdominal wall. These abdominal wall collaterals are best seen using a linear transducer.

A thickened lesser omentum can also indicate PHT. This sign is related to the dilatation of the omental and coronary veins and lymphatic congestion. Lesser omental thickness exceeding 1.7 times the aortic diameter on the sagittal scan indicates PHT [5,11].

Direct US visualization of the gastroesophageal varices using transabdominal scanning is rarely successful, even in pediatric patients, because of anatomic location and size of the veins; therefore, endoscopy is necessary to prove or to exclude the presence of these most important collaterals.

Reversed portal flow

Blood flows toward the liver in the splenoportal system (hepatopetal flow) in all normal subjects. Reversed or hepatofugal flow is considered a specific sign of increased portal pressure in PHT. Flow away from the liver in the splenic and superior mesenteric veins is a sign of increased intrahepatic resistance (Fig. 9), a rare finding seen only in advanced cases of liver disease. Reversed flow can be present in only one intrahepatic portal vein branch and can normalize depending on the patient's hepatic status after treatment. With continuous US observation, biphasic flow can sometimes be seen in the portal vein because of respiratory pressure effects [14].

Hepatic vein waveforms

The normal hepatic vein (HV) waveform is triphasic in healthy subjects because of variations of the central venous pressure during the cardiac cycle. This pattern changes in chronic liver disease and occurs in other conditions (cardiac congestion, tricuspid regurgitation). The HV waveforms are classified in three categories: normal triphasic (HV0), biphasic pattern or loss of the reverse component (HV1), and a flat waveform or pseudoportal waveform (HV2). The loss of the triphasic pattern is not a specific sign of cirrhosis or PHT; however, the occurrence of the biphasic and flat patterns is significantly higher in cirrhotic patients [15].

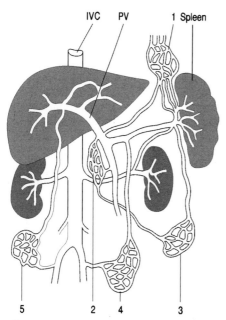

Fig. 7. Portosystemic collaterals in portal hypertension. The most important sites of portosystemic collaterals are shown. (1) Gastroesophageal. (2) Splenorenal. (3) Paracolic. (4) Pelvic. (5) Abdominal wall and paraumbilical veins. IVC, inferior vena cava; PV, portal vein. (*Adapted from* Harkanyi Z, Morvay Z, editors. Ultraszonografia. Budapest: Minerva; 2002. p. 107; with permission.)

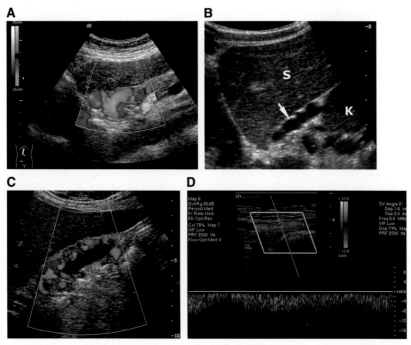

Fig. 8. Portal hypertension: collateral veins. (*A*) Sagittal color Doppler image shows a dilated left gastric or coronary vein. (*B*) Splenorenal varices (*arrow*) are sometimes visible by gray-scale scanning. S, spleen; K, kidney. (*C*) Color Doppler image shows gallbladder varices. If 2D image shows a thickened gall bladder wall, color Doppler can prove the presence of collaterals. (*D*) Duplex Doppler image showing a patent paraumbilical vein with hepatofugal flow.

Quantitative ultrasound evaluation of portal hypertension

In the past decades, several parameters have been suggested for the quantification of portal flow in healthy subjects and in patients who have liver disease (Table 3). It must be mentioned that the numbers published in the literature are valid for adult populations and few pediatric standards have been documented.

The size of the main portal vein can be measured with high accuracy. At a certain stage of PHT the central portal system is dilated. There is a poor correlation between the size of the portal vein and portal pressure, however, because the size of the portal veins is highly dependent on the blood volume shunted toward systemic veins (IVC and SVC). The sensitivity of portal vein size measurements alone is therefore insufficient to establish the diagnosis of PHT [10,16,17].

The size of the portal and superior mesenteric and splenic veins changes during respiration in normal subjects. Using good temporal resolution US systems, the size variations can be seen and

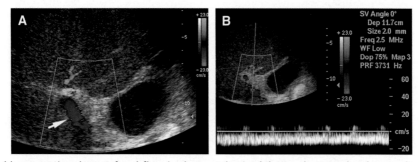

Fig. 9. Portal hypertension: hepatofugal flow in the portal vein. (*A*) 2D color Doppler shows color flow within the portal vein (*arrow*) is directed away from the transducer. Reversed flow in the portal vein is a specific sign of PHT. (*B*) Duplex Doppler shows the Doppler spectrum is below the baseline.

Table 3: **Quantitative evaluation of portal hypertension**

Parameter	Normal values	Changes in PHT	Ref.
Portal vein velocity	16–20.4 cm/sec	Decreases	[5,11]
Portal vein volume flow	648 ± 186 mL/min	Decreases	[8]
Venous pulsatility index (VPI)	0.48 ± 0.31	Decreases	[17]
Congestion index (CI)	0.07	Decreases	[20]
RI – hepatic artery	0.5–0.7	Decreases	[12]

measured. Lack of normal caliber change is suggestive of PHT, but this sign is unfortunately not sensitive enough to predict elevated portal pressure [10,18]. A recent study shows the same observation on the wall of the intrahepatic portion of the inferior vena cava. The IVC diameter decreases during deep inspiration in normal subjects, and this change is diminished in cirrhotic patients because of the stiffness of the liver parenchyma [19].

Mean and peak portal flow velocity can be measured by duplex US. The portal flow velocity depends on many factors, including the presence, type, and location of the portosystemic collaterals, the actual volume of blood shunting toward the IVC and SVC, and the severity of the parenchymal liver disease. The patient should be in a fasting state and multiple Doppler samples should be taken during breathholding. By measuring a large number of cirrhotic patients it was possible to document decreased mean flow velocity compared with healthy subjects. There is an overlap between the two groups, however, and the portal velocity analysis cannot allow the diagnosis of PHT in individual cases [2,20]. In addition, hyperdynamic circulation can occur in PHT, in which case increased flow velocity (and volume) is measured.

Portal volume flow in the main portal vein can be measured using Doppler methods with limited accuracy. The volume flow is calculated in mL/min based on the measurements of the mean flow velocity and the cross-sectional area of the portal vein. The errors of these two independent measurements are not negligible for technical and methodologic reasons, and added errors are reflected in the results. Because the data published show a wide variability according to different investigators, methods, and study populations, the clinical significance of this measurement is limited.

Calculated parameters of portal flow, such as the congestion index and venous pulsatility index, can also be used in adult and pediatric patients for the characterization of the actual hemodynamic status of the patient.

The venous pulsatility index (VPI) is calculated the same way as RI in arteries (Vmax−Vmin/Vmax) and normal values have been established [21–23].

VPI decreases in chronic liver disease; unfortunately there is again an overlap between healthy subjects and study groups. Nevertheless, it is a simple measurement that can be performed with good reproducibility.

The congestion index (CI) is defined as the ratio of cross-sectional area of the portal vein (cm^2) and the blood flow velocity (cm/sec). The vessel size increases and the flow velocity decreases in chronic liver disease, so the ratio decreases with PHT [24].

The meal test is another interesting way to examine portal flow changes as documented in the literature [25]. After eating (or preferably after the ingestion of a standardized meal), portal flow velocity and flow volume are increased by approximately 20% in healthy subjects. In patients who have chronic liver disorders, there is little or no increase. Postprandial flow increase occurs also in the HA.

The enlargement of the HA is a usual finding in cirrhosis. Decrease of blood flow in the portal system is compensated with higher flow in the HA. Elevated RI can be measured in the HA in patients who have chronic liver disease compared with healthy subjects [26].

In a large series of patients who have cirrhosis, the portocaval pressure gradient showed a weak correlation with measured US parameters [17]. From this and other studies it can be concluded that the clinical value of these measurements is limited by methodologic and pathophysiologic considerations.

Although the parameters mentioned have limitations as individual measurements, they can be applied in clinical settings and may be useful in following patients over time to assess for hemodynamic changes. These evaluations are most reliable if the US examination is performed on the same US system and by the same observer.

Endoscopic and other radiologic imaging methods in portal hypertension

Direct visualization of gastrointestinal varices is possible by endoscopy, endoscopic sonography, and endoluminal US. All these methods are

sensitive and accurate in showing the most danger-
ous source of GI hemorrhage. In contrast to endoscopy, US techniques are able to detect vessels under
the mucosal surface. The major limitation of these
modalities is their invasiveness, and sedation is required to perform the examination.

Multislice CT (MSCT) and MR imaging play important roles in the diagnosis and also in the follow-up of patients who have PHT. The inherent
limitations of US (bowel gas, obscured regions, lack
of cooperation in small children, operator depen-
dency) are well known, and CT or MR imaging is indicated in questionable cases.

MSCT represents a major advance in imaging
the liver and the hepatic vessels. Within a rapid
scanning time it is possible to image the liver parenchyma, the hepatic vessels, and any collaterals.
The 3D and multiplanar representation of the vol-
umetric CT data improves interpretation and is
readily understood by referring physicians. The
reproducibility of the studies is excellent. MSCT
demonstrates the portal system and abnormal
shunts with excellent spatial resolution in cirrhotic patients [27]. Limitations of CT are that it
gives no information on blood flow direction, it
uses ionizing radiation, and that contrast injection
is necessary [2].

MR imaging has a great potential in liver imaging, including the diagnosis of PHT. MR imaging
provides anatomic and functional data without
ionizing radiation on patients suffering from liver
disease and PHT, similar to US. Flow parameters determined by MR imaging are different in cirrhotic
patients compared with normal subjects [28]. Scanning time is longer compared with CT and US, and
it is the most expensive of all three methods. MR angiography is an optimal method for visualization of
surgical shunts (Fig. 10). Quantitative MR angiography of the splenoportal system has not been used
widely because of current technical limits, and
validation of the measurements has yet to be
established [2].

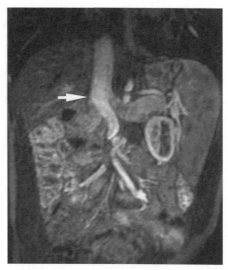

Fig. 10. Patent surgical mesocaval shunt on MR imaging. Although US can prove the patency of the surgical shunts, overlying bowel gas sometimes limits
visualization. MR imaging study shows a patent shunt
(*arrow*) 15 years after the operation.

TIPS provides a communication between the
right portal vein and the middle hepatic vein, to decompress the portal system (Fig. 11). Color Doppler is essential in the pretreatment evaluation and
also in the follow-up of patients after the TIPS procedure. Duplex Doppler is able to measure actual
flow velocity in the stent before and after the shunt.
Absolute velocity data can indicate stent stenosis
and also narrowing of the hepatic vein beyond
the stent. An in-stent venous velocity of more than
50 cm/sec indicates stenosis [29]. Stent dysfunction
can also be suspected using simple VPI measurement without angle corrected velocity measurement [30]. In cases of complete obstruction, no
flow is detected in the shunt.

Surgical portosystemic shunts are performed with
decreasing frequency because of their short-term

Treatment of portal hypertension and ultrasound imaging

Treatment options are determined by the type and
degree of PHT (Box 2). The most widespread way
of treatment is still endoscopically-guided sclerotherapy of gastroesophageal varices.

TIPS has become an effective treatment option in
cases of intrahepatic PHT in adults but is less frequently used in pediatric patients. The main application of TIPS in pediatric PHT is to provide enough
time to prepare the patient for liver transplantation,
if needed.

Box 2: Treatment options in portal hypertension

- Sclerotherapy
- Transjugular intrahepatic portosystemic shunt (TIPS)
- Surgical portosystemic shunts

  Porto-caval
  Meso-caval
  Distal spleno-renal
  Porto-mesenteric
  Spleno-pulmo

- *Drug therapy*

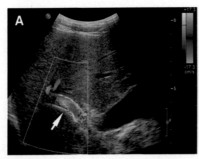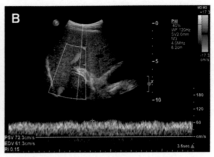

Fig. 11. Transjugular intrahepatic portosystemic shunt (TIPS). (A) Color Doppler image shows the stent (arrow) between the right portal vein and the hepatic vein. (B) Duplex Doppler confirms that the shunt is patent.

dangers and long-term problems. Currently the mesocaval shunt with a jugular graft interposed between the superior mesenteric vein and the inferior vena cava is the most common. Other types are distal or proximal splenorenal shunt, ilio-meso-caval shunt, and direct portocaval shunt. In cases of pre-hepatic-type PHT, a meso-portal procedure can be performed, if SMV is patent. Color Doppler and duplex US in experienced hands usually are able to prove the patency of these shunts [31]. If overlying bowel gas obscures direct US visualization of the shunts, MR angiography can be used.

Drug (medical) therapy is also used in the pediatric population suffering from PHT, though the results are contradictory and monitoring of the effect is difficult.

Summary

Sonography remains an optimal method in the evaluation of portal hypertension in pediatric patients. Color Doppler imaging provides good sensitivity flow detection in the portal venous system and also allows anatomic and functional analysis of the hepatic veins and hepatic artery even in small infants and children. The qualitative signs of portal hypertension should be searched for carefully. The clinical value of quantitative signs of PHT is limited by pathophysiologic and methodical considerations. Endoscopy, CT, and MR imaging are usually excellent complementary methods to US. They are invasive (endoscopy), costly, and less available than sonography. Color Doppler is also an essential method in the follow-up of patients who have an established diagnosis of PHT and also after various treatments.

References

[1] Franchis R. Evolving consensus in portal hypertension. Report of the Baveno IV consensus workshop on methodology of diagnosis and therapy in portal hypertension. J Hepatol 2005; 43:167–76.

[2] Vilgrain V. Ultrasound of diffuse liver disease and portal hypertension. In: Baert AL, Derchi LE, Grenier N, editors. Ultrasound. Categorical course ECR 2002 [syllabus]. Heidelberg: Springer; 2002. p. 91–105.

[3] Dahiya N. Liver and biliary tract. In: Khurana A, Dahiya N, editors. 3D and 4D ultrasound. A text and atlas. New Delhi: Jaypee Medical Publishers; 2004. p. 12–38.

[4] Albrecht T, Blomley MJ, Cosgrove DO, et al. Non-invasive diagnosis of hepatic cirrhosis by transit-time analysis of an ultrasound contrast agent. Lancet 1999;. 8;353(9164):1579–83.

[5] Siegel MJ. Liver. In: Siegel MJ, editor. Pediatric sonography. 3rd edition. Philadelphia: Lippincott Williams and Wilkins; 2002. p. 213–73.

[6] Harkanyi Z, Temesi M, Varga GY. Duplex ultrasonography in portal vein thrombosis. Surg Endosc 1989;3:79–81.

[7] Kim JH, Lee YS, Kim SH, et al. Does umbilical vein catheterization lead to portal venous thrombosis? Prospective US evaluation in 100 neonates. Radiology 2001;219:645–50.

[8] Gallego C, Miralles M, Marín C, et al. Congenital hepatic shunts. Radiographics 2004;24:755–72.

[9] Brawn BP, Abu-Youseff M, Farmer R, et al. Doppler sonography: a non-invasive method for evaluation of hepatic venoocclusive disease. Am J Roentgenol 1990;154:721–4.

[10] Vilgrain V, Lebrec D, Meno Y, et al. Comparison between ultrasonographic signs and degree of portal hypertension in patients with cirrhosis. Gastrointest Radiol 1990;15:218–22.

[11] Patriquin H, Lafortune M, Burns PN, et al. Duplex Doppler examination in portal hypertension: technique and anatomy. Am J Roentgenol 1987;149:71–6.

[12] Wachsberg RH, Simmons MZ. Coronary vein diameter and flow direction in patients with portal hypertension: evaluation with duplex sonography and correlation with variceal bleeding. Am J Roentgenol 1994;162:637–41.

[13] Ohnishi K, Sato S, Saito M, et al. Clinical and portal hemodynamic features in cirrhotic

patients having large spontaneous splenorenal and/or gastrorenal shunt. Am J Gastroenterol 1986;81:450.

[14] Wachsberg RH, Bahramipour P, Sofocleous CT, et al. Hepatofugal flow in the portal venous system: pathophysiology, imaging findings, and diagnostic pitfalls. Radiographics 2002; 22:123–40.

[15] Bolondi L, Bassi SL, Gaiani S, et al. Liver cirrhosis: changes of Doppler waveform of hepatic veins. Radiology 1991;178:513–6.

[16] Lafortune M, Marleau D, Breton G, et al. Portal venous measurements in portal hypertension. Radiology 1984;151:27.

[17] Haag K, Rossle M, Ochs A, et al. Correlation of duplex sonography findings and portal pressure in 375 patients with portal hypertension. Am J Roentgenol 1999;172:631–5.

[18] Zoli M, Dondi C, Marchesini G, et al. Splanchnic vein measurements in patients with liver cirrhosis: a case control study. J Ultrasound Med 1985; 4:641.

[19] Kitamura H, Kobayashi C. Impairment of change in diameter of the hepatic portion of the inferior vena cava: a sonographic sign of liver fibrosis or cirrhosis. J Ultrasound Med 2005;24:355–9.

[20] Zoli M, Marchesini G, Cordiani MR, et al. Echo-Doppler measurement of splanchnic vein blood flow in control and cirrhotic subjects. J Clin Ultrasound 1986;14:429–35.

[21] Wachsberg RH, Needleman L, Wilson DJ. Portal vein pulsatility in normal and cirrhotic adults without cardiac disease. J Clin Ultrasound 1995;23:3–15.

[22] Gallix BP, Taurel P, Dauzat M, et al. Flow pulsatility in the portal venous system: a study of Doppler sonography in healthy adults. Am J Roentgenol 1997;169:141–4.

[23] Barakat M. Portal vein pulsatility and spectral width changes in patients with portal hypertension: relation to the severity of liver disease. Br J Radiol 2002;75:417–21.

[24] Moriyasu F, Nishida O, Ban N, et al. "Congestion index" of the portal vein. Am J Roentgenol 1986; 146:735–9.

[25] Iwao T, Toyonaga A, Oho K, et al. Postprandial splanchnic hemodynamic response in patients with cirrhosis of the liver: evaluation with "triple-vessel" duplex US. Radiology 1996;201:711–5.

[26] Joynt LK, Platt JF, Rubin JM, et al. Hepatic artery resistance in cirrhosis before and after standard meal in subjects with diseased and healthy livers. Radiology 1995;196:489–92.

[27] Kang HK, Jeong YY, Choi JH, et al. Three-dimensional multi-detector row CT portal venography in the evaluation of portosystemic collateral vessels in liver cirrhosis. Radiographics 2002; 22:1053–61.

[28] Annet L, Materne R, Danse E. Hepatic flow parameters measured with MR imaging and Doppler US: correlations with degree of cirrhosis and portal hypertension. Radiology 2003; 229:409–14.

[29] Dodd GD III, Zajko AB, Orons PD, et al. Detection of transjugular intrahepatic portosystemic shunt dysfunction: value of duplex Doppler sonography. Am J Roentgenol 1995;164:1119–24.

[30] Sheiman RG, Vrachliotis T, Brophy DP, et al. Transmitted cardiac pulsations as an indicator of transjugular intrahepatic portosystemic shunt function: initial observations. Radiology 2002; 224:225–30.

[31] Lafortune M, Patriquin H, Pomier G, et al. Hemodynamic changes in portal circulation after portosystemic shunts: use of duplex sonography in 43 patients. Am J Roentgenol 1987;149:701–6.

ELSEVIER
SAUNDERS

Renal Failure in Neonates, Infants, and Children: The Role of Ultrasound

Michael Riccabona, MD

Renal failure is a serious, acute or chronic, reversible or irreversible, total or partial loss of excretory renal function with potentially deleterious sequelae, that unresolved may lead to dialysis or the need for renal transplantation. Pathophysiologically, there are three major causes:

- **Intrinsic RF with a disease process affecting the kidney itself**
- **Postrenal RF, usually secondary to obstructive uropathy**
- **Prerenal RF secondary to a systemic or extra-renal disease without an essential intrinsic kidney problem**

There are some situations in which more than one aspect is present or otherwise cannot be strictly classified according to these categories: systemic lupus erythematosus (SLE) with renal involvement and RF; hemolytic uremic syndrome (HUS) with RF secondary to bacterial or viral toxins and tubular congestion by hemolysis; hepatorenal syndrome; renal perfusion restriction in severe (bilateral) renal artery stenosis (RAS); traumatic renal vascular injury (tear, dissection, embolus); or crush kidneys with RF caused by tubular obstruction by myoglobin.

Clinically one can observe increased blood pressure and oliguria or anuria. Polyuria may precede or follow these stages, producing so-called "polyuric RF." Additionally there may be more or less generalized edema secondary to fluid overload or protein deficiency. Diagnosis is based on laboratory findings with elevated serum creatinine levels, electrolyte disturbances, low protein or albumin levels, and metabolic disturbances (such as acidosis). Additional symptoms or findings may be secondary to fluid overload (eg, hypertension, cardiomegaly and cardiac insufficiency, ascites, or pleural effusion) and metabolic problems (eg, tachypnea in severe acidosis).

Treatment options vary depending on the underlying condition, with supportive measures such as fluid and electrolyte balancing and hemofiltration being common. Treating systemic conditions and restoring circulation is necessary to overcome prerenal RF, and relief of obstruction is the treatment in postrenal RF. Intrinsic RF in general offers fewer

Department of Radiology, Division of Pediatric Radiology, University Hospital, LKH A–8036 Graz, Auenbruggenplatz, Austria
E-mail address: michael.riccabona@meduni-graz.at

doi:10.1016/j.cult.2006.05.004

treatment options, such as diet and fluid balance, antibiotics (in post- or parainfectious GN), steroids in some GN entities or nephritic and nephrotic syndrome (NS), and cytotoxic or immunosuppressive medication (eg, cyclophosphamide or cyclosporine in some forms of GN or NS).

In RF the role of imaging (and of US in particular) is initially to help differentiate acute from chronic and prerenal from postrenal or intrinsic RF. In some conditions, US can offer a treatment approach (eg, PCN, placing central lines for monitoring and dialysis), can assess the kidney during follow-up (eg, assessment of the amount of dilatation or by serial evaluation of renal perfusion using Doppler sonography [DS]), and can help establish the histologic diagnosis by offering a safe biopsy approach. US may also be helpful in evaluation of complications during the course of renal disease, to follow renal development and growth after recovery, or to check for sequelae and progression of a chronic disease under long-term treatment.

As this review focuses on pediatric US, several specific aspects important for diagnosis in neonates, infants, and children have to be mentioned. The neonatal kidney is still immature and thus on US appears different from a normal adult kidney. Normal creatinine levels change with age (normal in newborns, <0.5 mg/dL) because of increasing renal maturation, different metabolism, and growing body size. Different diseases occur than in adults: vascular disease is rare, although congenital malformations with renal hypodysplasia or autosomal recessive polycystic kidney disease (ARPKD) with early progression are more important in this age group. Sensitivity to radiation is higher in children, thus radiation-sparing imaging is even more important than in adults. Communication is different and there may be reduced patient cooperation. The different physiology and the different tissue composition (less fat and fibrous components) and the small size, different anatomic relations, and higher heart and respiration rates need technically different imaging equipment (high temporal and spatial resolution, different transducers) and cause different imaging appearances. All of these factors necessitate adapted imaging algorithms. This requires special knowledge and training and a dedicated infrastructure, because infants require different handling than do adults (eg, swaddling facilities, breastfeeding room, pacifiers, heating, and place for accompanying or assisting persons).

The aim of this article is to briefly list the various imaging modalities applicable in pediatric RF, to reflect on the task of imaging in infants and children with RF, and then to discuss the potential of US in pediatric RF with special regard to effective use of imaging.

Imaging modalities

Imaging is primarily based on US, supplemented by plain film, fluoroscopy, scintigraphy, and MR imaging in specific conditions and queries.

Ultrasound is the generally accepted basic imaging tool in RF. For a long time, however, US was seen as a "roughly orienting" method that allowed for depiction of collecting system dilatation or urinary tract malformations, but it did not offer any more detailed information. This started to change initially with the advent of DS, then color Doppler sonography (CDS) and particularly amplitude-coded CDS (aCDS). These tools enabled assessment of renal perfusion and helped in differentiating various conditions, such as prerenal failure, focal renal lesions, or renal vein thrombosis [1–3]. Gray-scale imaging was then improved by the introduction of high-resolution US, image compounding, and harmonic imaging [3–6]. Upcoming techniques, such as intravenous US contrast agents, together with refined sonographic contrast depiction capabilities, will further enhance US potential, making US a comprehensive, noninvasive, portable imaging tool that allows for anatomic and functional (ie, perfusion, vesicoureteral reflux [VUR]) evaluation of the urinary tract [3,7–12]. US thus has become the major imaging tool for pediatric RF.

Plain films are rarely useful or indicated in patients who have RF. Evaluation of systemic sequelae, assessment of central line position, or the initial diagnostic evaluation, however, often require a chest film, and diagnosing some underlying conditions such as urolithiasis still may require a plain film [13]. Note that film speed and exposure need to be adapted to age and weight and that digital radiography may lack sufficient resolution, particularly in neonates and infants. Fluoroscopy is applied in VCUG for diagnosing PUV or VUR with associated renal dysplasia and in angiography or interventional procedures, such as PCN [14–17].

The value of CT is limited in the pediatric urinary tract and in particular in RF, because RF is a contraindication for the use of intravenous contrast material required in most pediatric urinary tract queries [18–20]. The primary indication for CT in the pediatric urinary tract is major trauma or work-up of renal tumors and tumorlike lesions, usually not presenting with RF and as such beyond the scope of this article.

The two other major imaging players in RF are scintigraphy and, increasingly, MR imaging. Static renal scintigraphy (Tc^{99m} DMSA) is used for evaluating overall and split renal function. Diuretic dynamic renal scintigraphy (Tc^{99m} MAG3) is considered the gold standard for assessment and grading of obstructing uropathy. MRI has successfully been introduced into pediatric uroradiology [21–28]. New technical refinements and sequence modifications promise to widen the potential of MR urography (MRU) to become a comprehensive "all in one" imaging tool, offering not only anatomic assessment but additionally providing detailed and quantitative functional information. MR contrast material may be given in RF because of its reduced nephrotoxicity, allowing assessment of renal perfusion and residual function. Diffusion-weighted imaging and new intracellular contrast materials promise to open yet unexplored diagnostic fields for imaging diagnosis and prognostic assessment.

The use of imaging in typical pediatric diseases and common clinical queries

Severe pediatric RF is a rare but serious and life-threatening condition that needs urgent diagnosis and treatment. The differential diagnoses of neonatal RF include [29–35]:

- Intrinsic renal diseases, such as severe urinary tract infection, renal vein thrombosis, hypoxic and toxic renal parenchymal damage (including treatment- or drug-induced), congenital hypodysplasia, bilateral renal agenesis, ARPKD, congenital NS, syndromatic nephropathies, and neonatal GN
- Postrenal problems caused by bilateral severe obstructing uropathy (ie, PUV, megaureter with uretero-vesicle junction obstruction, and uretero-pelvic junction obstruction)
- Prerenal RF caused by systemic problems, such as septicemia and multiorgan system failure, heart disease (particularly PDA and aortic coarctation), hypotension and hypovolemia (eg, after placental bleeding or uterine rupture), or dehydration and hyperviscosity

In older children, RF may evolve because of an underlying chronic condition, some of them

syndromal or hereditary (eg, reflux nephropathy, [RNP]), juvenile nephronophthisis, or Alport syndrome), and subsequent chronic RF is more common. Additional intrinsic renal diseases that may cause acute RF entities have to be considered: HUS, NS, para- or postinfectious GN, tubular renal acidosis (or oxalosis and cystinosis) with consecutive progressive nephrocalcinosis, various tubulopathies, renal involvement in systemic diseases such as in Henoch-Schönlein disease or SLE, or toxic- and drug-induced RF (ie, herbs and fungus, chemotherapy, antibiotics, or intravenous iodinated contrast agents) [20,36–42]. Furthermore, acute obstruction caused by urinary tract calculus or an abdominal tumor, renal destruction by tumors, or chronic infections, such as xanthogranulomatous pyelonephritis, and traumatic RF (eg, bladder rupture, crush kidney, or vascular injury) need to be mentioned as rare causes for pediatric RF to complete the list. Looking at all these entities, it becomes obvious that a thorough and detailed discussion of these diseases would fill a book and thus is beyond the scope of this brief overview. Most nephropathies, however, have similar or even identical imaging appearances. The author focuses only on modern US features in typical neonatal and pediatric conditions.

Intrinsic renal conditions

Neonatal presentation of RF is often suggested prenatally; the correct diagnosis of the most common renal causes, however, is eventually established after birth. ARPKD and congenital NS ("of the Finnish type") or—less often—neonatal GN are the most common causes, with some more or less typical imaging features. In general, ARPKD exhibits the typical "pepper and salt" appearance of the parenchyma of an enlarged and hyperechoic kidney, usually with no or just a few tiny cysts seen (Fig. 1) [32–35]. Neonatal GN and NS also present with an enlarged kidney and some alteration of the parenchymal echo pattern; no specific features are known, although some differences in corticomedullary

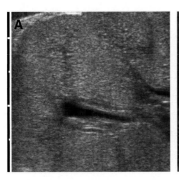 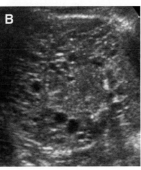

Fig. 1. (*A*) Transverse sonogram of neonatal ARPKD shows echogenic parenchyma without any corticomedullary differentiation. (*B*) Transverse sonogram in an infant who had syndromatic cystic renal parenchymal disease shows multiple parenchymal cysts and absent corticomedullary differentiation.

differentiation and in the amount and pattern of echogenicity changes have been noted to be more common in some diseases [34,35,43]. Even DS findings (reduced peripheral vasculature on aCDS, increased or decreased RI or velocities on DDS) are nonspecific and correspond better with renal function (degree of renal failure, modulated by therapeutic aspects such as fluid load, drugs, blood pressure modulation, and heart rate) than with the underlying disease entity. This is also valid in other forms of GN or NS as seen in older children, such as para- and postinfectious GN, Henoch-Schönlein nephritis and IgA-nephropathy, lupus nephritis, or (familial) NS (Fig. 2) [3,38,40,41]. Usually kidney size is enlarged or normal, and US appearance depends on the relative echogenicity of the cortex and the parenchyma. Corticomedullary differentiation thus depends on whether both or only one of these structures is affected, how much each of them are affected and may be increased or decreased, or sometimes are even normal in mild disease. The US appearances are thus rather nonspecific, and the value of US in these patients is not to specify a certain disease (although some suggestions concerning the underlying disease may be achievable), but rather to (1) rule out other potential causes for RF, (2) assess the amount of pleural effusion or ascites and intravascular fluid load for balancing supportive measures, and (3) assess extrarenal disease aspects.

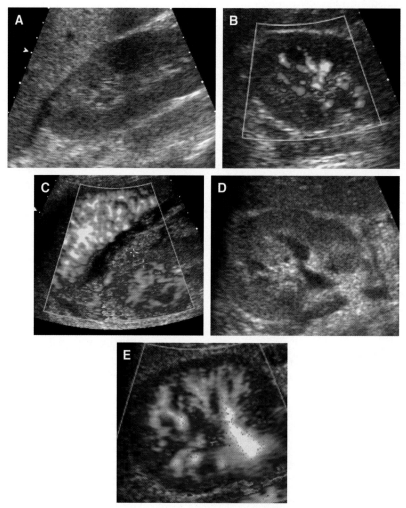

Fig. 2. (*A*) Unspecific renal parenchymal changes in severe Lupus nephritis. (*B*) Significantly reduced peripheral renal perfusion in aRF shown by aCDS. (*C*) Reduced perfusion of the renal cortex (*cursors*) becomes even more obvious when compared with the aCDS vascularity of the adjacent spleen. (*D*) Transverse sonogram through a right kidney in NS. (*E*) Peripherally reduced vasculature on aCDS (halo sign) indicating restricted peripheral renal perfusion.

Renal vein thrombosis

Renal vein thrombosis mostly occurs in neonates who have adrenal gland hemorrhage, coagulopathies, femoral central lines, or dehydration and polyglobulic syndrome [3,44–46]. Note that unilateral renal vein thrombosis usually presents with hypertension and hematuria and should not lead to global RF except for single systems or coexisting impairment of the other kidney. In neonates, thrombosis usually starts in the peripheral veins, only gradually growing into the central veins, behaving similarly to tumor thrombi (Fig. 3A). In older children, extrarenal origin of thrombosis or a primary thrombus of the major renal vein is more common. The basic and often single imaging tool is US, demonstrating a large, swollen, and hyperechoic kidney with undifferentiated parenchyma (Fig. 3B). On CDS, renal vein color signals are missing in the affected veins, although they may be demonstrable in patent central veins. DDS shows increased

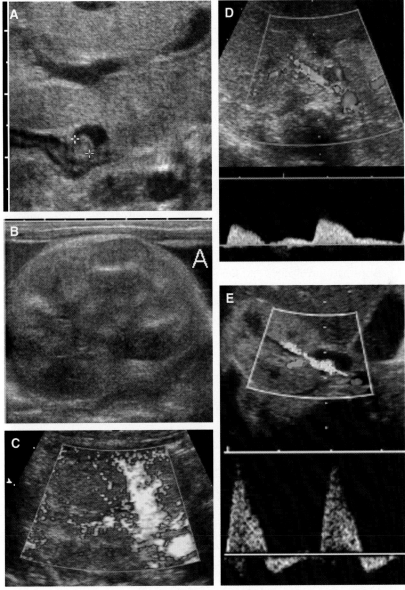

Fig. 3. (*A*) Transverse sonogram showing renal vein thrombus (*between cursors*) reaching into the IVC. (*B*) Longitudinal image showing a swollen kidney with hazy corticomedullary differentiation in neonatal renal vein thrombosis. Note the secondary ascites (A). (*C*) Longitudinal aCDS image demonstrates regionally diminished perfusion in partial/peripheral neonatal renal vein thrombosis. CDS with DDS trace depicts the (*D*) increasingly reduced and then (*E*) reversed diastolic flow with elevated RI.

arterial resistance with high resistive indices (RI) and low or missing diastolic flow (Fig. 3C–E). On follow-up—even with some treatment success—one often observes shrinkage of the kidney with diffusely abnormal echo pattern of the parenchyma and reduced perfusion. These changes sometimes only become apparent over time, as a lack of age-concordant renal growth with contralateral compensatory renal hypertrophy. Usually no other imaging is needed except for tumor conditions, in which MR imaging (or CT) and MR angiography (MRA) are performed for overall assessment and staging and preoperative planning.

Congenital hypodysplasia

Congenital hypodysplasia (with RF) may be somewhat difficult to diagnose. Only the most severe forms (eg, bilateral multicystic dysplastic kidney) are easily and often prenatally recognizable, though sometimes not compatible with extrauterine life. As described by the name, the affected kidneys usually are small and present an altered echotexture with reduced corticomedullary differentiation and increased echogenicity; cysts of varying size may be present (Fig. 4A). The amount of these changes depends on the degree of dysplasia, however, and pure hypoplasia may initially even exhibit normal US features, with the kidney size initially ranging within normal limits [32–34]. Only over time does the size deficit perhaps become obvious and then may eventually correspond to developing and progressive chronic RF. This entity may be difficult to be distinguished from RNP (a term that is increasingly under discussion). The underlying renal pathology in RNP usually is a combination of coexisting congenital renal dysplasia with renal growth retardation and acquired renal damage caused by infection and scarring associated with VUR that may have vanished by the time of diagnosis (Fig. 4B). The "water hammer theory" for RNP is (postnatally) probably only valid in some patients

who have severe, long lasting, high pressure VUR usually associated with bladder dysfunction.

Hemolytic uremic syndrome

HUS is a condition in which acute RF is caused by toxins of a certain *Escherichia coli* strain affecting the renal cortical and glomerular capillaries causing vasculopathy, hemolysis, and thrombosis. It is a disease that may occur as familial or endemic (in certain areas and populations) and incidentally, preferably affecting young patients during early summer. Diagnosis is assumed in case of a recent, sometimes hemorrhagic enterocolitis with acute RF, thrombocytopenia, anemia, hypertension, and typical erythrocyte morphology on microscopy (fragmented cells called Burr cells or schistocytes), and is confirmed by culture results. Treatment options are restricted to symptomatic measures and renal replacement therapy. Prognosis varies; in a single event a good outcome is common. In prolonged, chronic, and recurrent disease, prognosis concerning renal functional outcome is poorer, though mortality has been nearly eradicated. US demonstrates bilaterally enlarged kidneys with a large, hyperechoic cortex and increased corticomedullary differentiation (Fig. 5A,B). RI is markedly increased (Fig. 5C), and aCDS exhibits diffusely reduced cortical perfusion with a marked uncolored peripheral halo [34,39–41]. Additionally, US examination may demonstrate regional bowel wall thickening and secondary signs of acute RF and bowel inflammation. During the course of the disease, improvement of DDS with gradually improving RI values precedes clinical improvement of renal function and thus may be useful for monitoring and for making therapy decisions.

Eventually US can help to establish the histologic diagnosis in intrinsic renal conditions producing RF, which may be essential for treatment decisions and prognostic estimation, by providing safe biopsy guidance [14–17,47–49]. Here US not only helps to guide the biopsy, thus increasing safety and

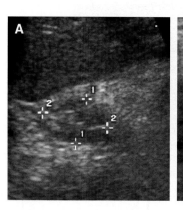
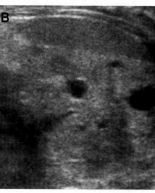

Fig. 4. (*A*) Transverse sonogram of the right kidney demonstrates a small kidney (*cursors*) with atypical parenchymal structure. (*B*) Transverse sonogram of a left kidney shows cystic defects in a neonatal kidney with increased echogenicity and reduced corticomedullary differentiation in "congenital RNP."

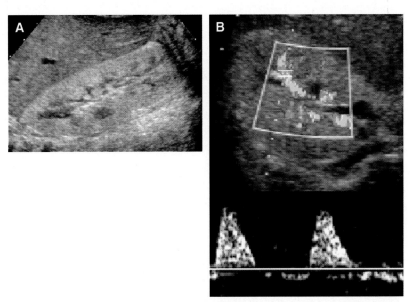

Fig. 5. (*A*) Longitudinal sonogram of an enlarged right kidney demonstrates the typical US appearance of an acutely affected kidney in HUS with increased cortical echogenicity and corticomedullary differentiation. (*B*) Transverse CDS with duplex tracing demonstrates the markedly reduced perfusion with reversed diastolic flow and increased RI.

enabling a satisfactory specimen harvest with a minimum of needle passes, but is also essential for postbiopsy monitoring and identification of postbiopsy complications, such as hemorrhage, urinary tract obstruction by clots, or postbiopsy arteriovenous fistula (AVF) (Fig. 6).

Postrenal conditions

In obstructing uropathy, all features of acute or chronic urinary tract obstruction may be observed. Acute obstruction (eg, by a ureteral calculus) usually exhibits little dilatation, as may severe obstruction

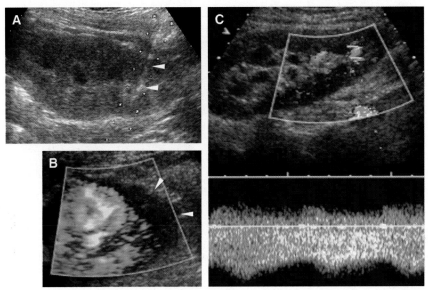

Fig. 6. (*A*) US-guided biopsy with the needle (*arrowheads*) passing into the lower pole of the left kidney as predefined by the dotted needle trace of the guiding device. (*B*) Postbiopsy hematoma on the lower pole of the left kidney (*arrowheads*), superiorly delineated by aCDS. (*C*) CDS depicts a postbiopsy AVF as shown by focal aliasing in the lower pole and elevated diastolic arterial flow.

with subsequently deteriorated renal function. US demonstration of dilatation of the renal collecting system or the ureter does not necessarily equal obstruction. To exhibit a severely dilated system, good urine production is needed and thus this finding may indirectly indicate persisting renal function [31,32]. Polyuria (polyuric phase of RF, stimulated diuresis, volume overload) and laxity of a collecting system (eg, in neonates or in infection) may cause some dilatation that should not be misinterpreted as urinary tract "obstruction." In these conditions RF only occurs in single obstructed systems or in bilateral disease (such as bilateral UPJO or PUV with bilateral obstructing or refluxing megaureter and renal dysplasia) (Fig. 7).

The role of US is to detect collecting system dilatation and to suggest the cause and the level of obstruction (urinary calculus, UPJO, accessory renal artery) (Fig. 8A,B). US may help to differentiate acute from chronic obstruction; in acute obstruction DDS may reveal an asymmetrically elevated RI at usually little dilatation and diffusely increased echogenicity of the enlarged and swollen kidney [3,44–46,50–53]. In this setting, modern US tools such as aCDS, DDS, and 3D US may become helpful. For example, the depiction of an ostial ureteral jet into the urinary bladder by CDS may demonstrate ureteral patency and the UVJ (see Fig. 7A); diffusely decreased (peripheral) renal perfusion on aCDS (halo sign) may hint toward more severe

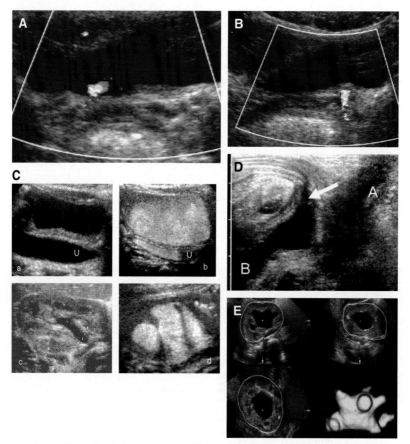

Fig. 7. (*A*) Transverse CDS through the lower pelvis and urinary bladder demonstrates a right ostial ureteric jet, with lack of depictable urine inflow into the bladder on the left side caused by a distal ureteral calculus. (*B*) The "twinkling sign": CDS demonstrates twinkling color signals within the distal ureter at the ureterovesical junction caused by a small distal ureteral calculus in the same patient as seen in (*A*). (*C*) Echo-enhanced urosonography (A). Initial longitudinal sonogram shows a dilated ureter (U) posterior to the urinary bladder (B). After instillation of Levovist into the prefilled urinary bladder, VUR is seen as echogenic material in the dilated distal ureter (U). Furthermore, the initially narrow renal pelvis of the corresponding kidney (C) becomes markedly dilated and filled with US contrast material (D), indicating high-grade VUR. (*D*) Longitudinal perineal US demonstrating PUV (*arrow*) with the typical dilated bladder neck appearance. B, bladder; A, anal canal. (*E*) 3D US in hydronephrosis: outlining of outer renal contour (*green line*) for volume calculation in three orthogonal sections, with deduction of the segmented dilated collecting system as visualized in the right lower box for estimation of renal parenchymal volume.

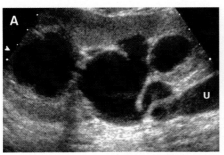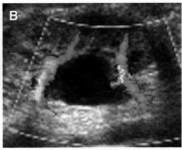

Fig. 8. (*A*) Longitudinal sonogram demonstrates marked dilatation of the collecting system with a kink at the pelviureteric junction and a megaureter (U). (*B*) Longitudinal CDS sonogram in a kidney with dilated renal pelvis depicts an additional renal artery crossing the ureteropelvic junction and potentially causing obstruction.

conditions; the "twinkling sign" on CDS improves detection of ureteral calculi (see Fig. 7B); perineal US may enable detection of a PUV (see Fig. 7C); echo-enhanced urosonography may enable differentiation of refluxing versus obstructing uropathy (see Fig. 7D); and relative renal parenchymal volume assessment by 3D US may help estimate split renal parenchymal size (see Fig. 7E) [3,4,6–12].

In severe obstruction or pyohydronephrosis, US is the ideal imaging modality to guide percutaneous nephrostomy (PCN), potentially complimented by fluoroscopy for comprehensive visualization of the entire collecting system anatomy and for detection of potential extravasations [10,14,15,17]. Note that indications for operation and PCN have changed over the past decade; now only severe conditions with acute threat to renal function or intractable urinary tract infection are considered indications for these invasive treatment options.

Prerenal conditions

Prerenal RF is defined by an extrarenal condition causing renal hypoperfusion and hypoxia. The most common causes are trauma with blood loss and shock or other causes of prolonged hypovolemia and hypoxia (eg, drowning, complicated operation, asphyxia, vascular injury) and cardiac disease or malformations, such as persisting duct of Botallo (patent ductus arteriosus) with left-to-right shunt, aortic coarctation, and heart failure. The US findings are nonspecific, demonstrating normal kidneys (particularly in early stages) or bilaterally swollen, often diffusely hyperechoic kidneys. Perfusion alterations on DS, such as decreased flow velocities with "pseudonormal" or elevated RI values, flattened systolic flow curves, and pathologically delayed systolic flow acceleration can be seen (Fig. 9). US is used to assess the degree of perfusion disturbance, to find or rule out other renal conditions, to evaluate the systemic changes of the underlying condition, such as free peritoneal or retroperitoneal fluid (in trauma),

cardiac function (by echocardiography), brain perfusion (by transfontanellar or transtemporal DDS), and to monitor renal perfusion as a prognostic indicator or for treatment guidance.

Renal transplantation

Increasingly, even small children who have terminal RF can now be treated by renal transplantation, with an improved long-term outcome and a better life quality compared with chronic dialysis, which may still be needed until a compatible transplant organ is available. Imaging in these children is primarily based on US. Initially, donor organs are evaluated by US before explantation. Then early postoperative surveillance uses serial US and DDS/CDS, particularly in evaluating transplant malfunction (eg, tubular necrosis, early rejection, vascular problems, and obstructed urinary drainage). Assessment of kidney size, renal parenchymal structure, and potential dilatation of the collecting system is mandatory, as is visualization of the main supplying vessels, including a DDS and aCDS assessment of renal perfusion. Furthermore, evaluation of the vascular anastomosis is desirable to depict stenoses or aneurysm formation (Fig. 10).

During later post-transplant phases, routine US investigations are performed to monitor renal growth and to detect early stages of potential rejection or (*Cyclosporine*-induced) vasculopathy, particularly if clinical and laboratory findings indicate a potential problem. In this scenario, transplant organ size changes are one of the most sensitive, though unspecific, signs to detect transplant disease. Additional findings in transplant disease are changed parenchymal echogenicity and corticomedullary differentiation, dilatation of the collecting system (in stenosis of ureteral anastomosis), increased RI values (in rejection and vasculopathy), flattened systolic flow acceleration (in renal artery stenosis, usually located near the anastomosis), regional venous flow turbulences (more likely in

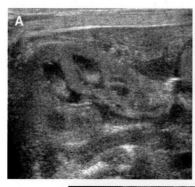

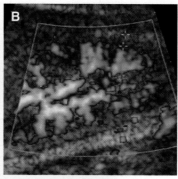

Fig. 9. (*A*) Normal gray scale appearance of a neonatal right kidney, with some surrounding edematous soft tissue. (*B*) aCDS demonstrates reduced peripheral vasculature (*cursors*) with a somewhat patchy pattern of vessel rarefaction. (*C*) CDS with duplex tracing shows an elevated RI with a reversed diastolic flow but a normal systolic flow profile.

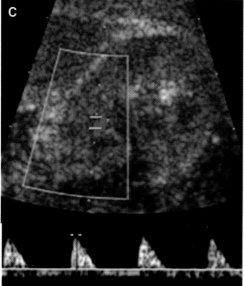

vasculopathy or partial renal vein thrombosis), AVF (after biopsies), and impaired peripheral perfusion demonstrated by reduced peripheral color signals on aCDS (usually in significant functional impairment) or regional lack of aCDS-depictable perfusion (in segmental infarction). US, however, (and scintigraphy and MR imaging) often remains nonspecific as to the disease entity, and US-guided transplant biopsy may become necessary for definitive diagnosis and further management decisions. Extrarenal complications, such as post-transplant lymphoproliferative disease, have to also be considered in long-term imaging follow-up of transplant patients.

Follow-up evaluation

Finally, follow-up is a critical aspect of managing patients who have acute or chronic RF. US serves as a follow-up tool, allowing for noninvasive monitoring of renal perfusion, evaluation of collecting system dilatation, and assessment of renal parenchymal growth. Even after renal transplantation or during dialysis, the original kidneys, the urinary bladder, and the renal transplant may develop disease that needs imaging, such as secondary cystic changes, malignancy, infection, or transplant malfunction. Other imaging modalities, such as VCUG, IVU, plain film, scintigraphy, or MRU, may be indicated for a complete work-up of the underlying condition, particularly preoperatively and in complex urogenital malformations. Similarly, following patients who have chronic RF also may require the use of other imaging modalities, such as plain film or MR imaging, for diagnosis of systemic sequelae or treatment complications, such as hypertension and cardiomyopathy or osteonecrosis during steroid treatment.

Summary

US is the ideal and often single imaging modality in infants and children who have acute or chronic RF. Modern US tools and US-guided renal biopsy offer extended diagnostic capabilities, eventually enabling a safe histologic definition of a nephropathy

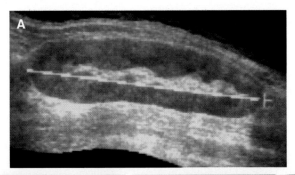

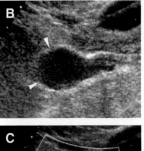

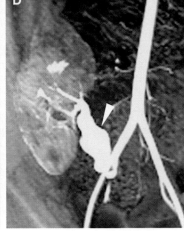

Fig. 10. (*A*) Extended field of view technique to properly cover the entire kidney for reliable length measurement not achievable by a conventional single US image, if a large organ is located close to the skin. (*B–D*) Aneurysm (*arrowheads*) of a venous patch at the anastomosis of the transplant's main renal artery, visualized by (*B*) conventional US and (*C*) CDS, confirmed by (*D*) MRA.

that cannot be sufficiently diagnosed by clinical, laboratory, and imaging findings. The imaging approach for children who have RF thus heavily relies on US as the primary imaging modality. It always starts with an initial US study (including DDS and CDS) to differentiate pre-, post-, or intrarenal origin of RF and to assess the severity of renal perfusion (and thus functional) impairment. Uncommonly, other imaging techniques, such as plain film, scintigraphy, or MR imaging are necessary for initial assessment and therapeutic decisions, depending on the initial US results, the general patient condition, and the underlying disease. Follow-up imaging assessment is primarily by US (focused on renal size, parenchyma, and perfusion), often complemented by scintigraphy (or, in the future, increasingly by MR imaging) to assess overall renal function and parenchymal scarring. Occasionally, specific diseases or complications may indicate additional imaging; some conditions may be diagnosed or managed by US-guided interventions.

Modern US techniques, a US facility and equipment adapted and suited for pediatric needs, specific knowledge, and education are compulsory to make the utmost use of the great potential of US. Children are not just small adults, but present specific diseases and different imaging appearances, and deserve special, focused, and skilled care.

References

[1] Riccabona M, Schwinger W, Ring E, et al. Amplitude coded color Doppler sonography in pediatric renal disease. Eur Radiol 2001;11:861–6.

[2] Riccabona M. Pediatric ultrasound. I. Abdomen. Eur Radiol 2001;11:2354–68.

[3] Riccabona M. Potential of modern sonographic techniques in paediatric uroradiology. Eur J Radiol 2002;43:110–21.

[4] Aytac SK, Ozcan H. Effect of color Doppler system on the twinkling sign associated with urinary tract calculi. J Clin Ultrasound 1999; 27:433–9.

[5] Bartram U, Darge K. Harmonic versus conventional ultrasound imaging of the urinary tract in children. Pediatr Radiol 2005;35:655–60.

[6] Cehfouh N, Grenier N, Higueret D. Characterization of urinary calculi: in vitro study of twinkling artifact revealed by color-flow sonography. Am J Radiol 1998;171:1055–60.

[7] Darge K, Tröger J, Duetting T, et al. Reflux in young patients: comparison of voiding US of the bladder and the retrovesical space with echoenhancement versus voiding cystourethrography for diagnosis. Radiology 1999;210:201–7.

[8] Darge K, Moeller RT, Trusen A, et al. Diagnosis of vesicoureteric reflux with low-dose contrast-enhanced harmonic ultrasound imaging. Pediatr Radiol 2005;35:73–8.

[9] Riccabona M, Uggowitzer M, Klein E, et al. Contrast enhanced color Doppler sonography in children and adolescents. J Ultrasound Med 2000;19:783–8.

[10] Riccabona M, Mache CJ, Lindbichler F. Echo-enhanced color Doppler cystosonography of vesico-ureteral reflux in children: improvement by stimulated acoustic emission. Acta Radiol 2003;44:18–23.

[11] Riccabona M, Fritz G, Ring E. Potential applications of three-dimensional ultrasound in the pediatric urinary tract: pictorial demonstration based on preliminary results. Eur Radiol 2003; 13:2680–7.

[12] Riccabona M, Fritz GA, Schollnast H, et al. Hydronephrotic kidney: pediatric three-dimensional US for relative renal size assessment–initial experience. Radiology 2005;236:276–83.

[13] Riccabona M, Lindbichler F, Sinzig M. Conventional imaging in paediatric uroradiology. Eur J Radiol 2002;43:100–9.

[14] Riccabona M, Sorantin E, Hausegger K. Imaging guided interventional procedures in paediatric uroradiology—a case-based overview. Eur J Radiol 2002;43:167–79.

[15] Riccabona M. Interventional uroradiology in paediatrics: a potpourri of diagnostic and therapeutic options. Minerva Pediatr 2004; 56:497–505.

[16] Riccabona M, Mache CJ, Dell'Acqua A, et al. Renal biopsy. In: Fotter R, editor. Pediatric uroradiology. Berlin–Heidelberg–New York: Springer; 2001. p. 272–4.

[17] Stanely P, Diamet MJ. Pediatric percutaneous nephrostomy: experience with 50 patients. J Urol 1986;135:1223–6.

[18] Marcos SK. Contrast media induced nephrotoxicity—questions and answers. Br J Radiol 1998; 71:357–65.

[19] Maudgil DD, McHugh K. The role of CT in modern pediatric uroradiology. Eur J Radiol 2002; 43:129–38.

[20] Murphy SW, Barrett BJ, Parfrey PS. Contrast nephropathy. J Am Soc Nephrol 2000;11:177–82.

[21] Avni FE, Nicaise N, Hall M, et al. The role of MR imaging for the assessment of complicated duplex kidneys in children: preliminary report. Pediatr Radiol 2001;31:215–23.

[22] Borthne A, Nordshus T, Reiseter T, et al. MR urography: the future gold standard in paediatric urogenital imaging? Pediatr Radiol 1999; 29:694–701.

[23] Borthne A, Pierre-Jerome C, Nordshus T, et al. MR urography in children: current status and future development. Eur Radiol 2000;10:503–11.

[24] Riccabona M, Simbrunner J, Ring E, et al. Feasibility of MR-urography in neonates and infants with anomalies of the upper urinary tract. Eur Radiol 2002;12:1442–50.

[25] Riccabona M. Pediatric MRU—its potential and its role in the diagnostic work-up of upper urinary tract dilatation in infants and children. World J Urol 2004;22:79–87.

[26] Rohrschneider WK, Haufe S, Wiesel M, et al. Functional and morphologic evaluation of congenital urinary tract dilatation by using combined static-dynamic MR urography: findings in kidneys with a single collecting system. Radiology 2002;224:683–94.

[27] Rohrschneider WK, Hoffend J, Becker K, et al. Combined static-dynamic MR urography for the simultaneous evaluation of morphology and function in urinary tract obstruction. I. Evaluation of the normal status in an animal model. Pediatr Radiol 2000;30:511–22.

[28] Sigmund G, Stoever B, Zimmerhackl LB, et al. RARE-MR-urography in the diagnosis of upper urinary tract abnormalities in children. Pediatr Radiol 1991;21:416–20.

[29] Bratton VS, Ellis EN, Seibert JT. Ultrasonographic findings in congenital nephrotic syndrome. Pediatr Nephrol 1990;4:515–6.

[30] Feitz WFJ, Cornellissen EAM, Blickman JG. Renal disease and renal failure. In: Carty H, Brunelle F, Stringer DA, et al, editors. 2nd edition, Imaging children, Vol. 1. Edinburgh-London-New York-Oxford-Philadelphia-St. Louis-Sydney-Toronto: Elsevier; 2005. p. 617–42.

[31] Gordon I, Barratt TM. Imaging the kidneys and urinary tract in the neonate with acute renal failure. Pediatr Nephrol 1987;1:321–9.

[32] Gordon I, Riccabona M. Investigating the newborn kidney—update on imaging techniques. Semin Neonatol 2003;8:269–78.

[33] Riccabona M, Ring E. Renal agenesis, dysplasia, hypoplasia and cystic diseases of the kidney. In: Fotter R, editor. Pediatric uroradiology. Berlin-Heidelberg-New York: Springer; 2001. p. 229–52.

[34] Riccabona M, Mache CJ, Dell'Aqua A, et al. Renal parenchymal disease. In: Fotter R, editor. Pediatric uroradiology. Berlin-Heidelberg-New York: Springer; 2001. p. 253–80.

[35] Ring E, Fotter R. The newborn with oligoanuria. In: Fotter R, editor. Pediatric uroradiology. Berlin-Heidelberg-New York: Springer; 2001. p. 313–20.

[36] Cameron JS. Lupus nephritis. J Am Soc Nephrol 1999;10:413–24.

[37] Chesney RW. The idiopathic nephrotic syndrome. Curr Opin Pediatr 1999;11:158–61.

[38] Gershen RS, Brody AS, Duffy LC, et al. Prognostic value of sonography in childhood nephrotic syndrome. Pediatr Nephrol 1994;8:76–8.

[39] Choyke PL, Grant EG, Hoffer FA, et al. Cortical echogenicity in the hemolytic uremic syndrome: clinical correlation. J Ultrasound Med 1988; 7:439–42.

[40] Garel L, Habib R, Babin C, et al. Hemolytic uremic syndrome. Diagnosis and prognostic value of ultrasound. Ann Radiol (Paris) 1983;26:169–74.

[41] Patriquin HB, O'Regan S, Robitaille P, et al. Hemolytic-uremic syndrome: intrarenal arterial Doppler patterns as a useful guide to therapy. Radiology 1989;172:625–8.

[42] Repetto HA. Epidemic hemolytic-uremic syndrome in children. Kidney Int 1997;52:1708–19.

[43] Salame H, Damry N, Vandenhoudt K, et al. The contribution of ultrasound for the differential diagnosis of congenital and infantile nephrotic syndrome. Eur Radiol 2003;13:2674–9.

[44] Errington ML, Hendry GM. The rare association of right adrenal haemorrhage and renal vein thrombosis diagnosed with duplex ultrasound. Pediatr Radiol 1995;25;157–8.

[45] Hibbert J, Howlett DC, Greenwood KL, et al. The ultrasound appearances of neonatal renal vein thrombosis. Br J Radiol 1997;70:1191–4.

[46] Wright NB, Blanch G, Walkinshaw S, et al. Antenatal and neonatal renal vein thrombosis: new ultrasonic features with high frequency transducers. Pediatr Radiol 1996;26:686–9.

[47] Gainza FJ, Minguela I, Lopez-Vidaur I, et al. Evaluation of complications due to percutaneous renal biopsy in allograft and native kidneys with color-coded Doppler sonography. Clin Nephrol 1995;43:303–8.

[48] Obek SS, Memis A, Killi R, et al. Image directed and color Doppler ultrasonography in the diagnosis of postbiopsy arteriovenous fistula of native kidneys. J Clin Ultrasound 1995;23:239–42.

[49] Riccabona M, Schwinger W, Ring E. Arteriovenous fistula after renal biopsy in children. J Ultrasound Med 1998;17:505–8.

[50] Kessler RM, Quevedo H, Lankau CA, et al. Obstructive vs. nonobstructive dilatation of the renal collecting system in children: distinction with duplex sonography. Am J Roentgenol 1993;160:353–7.

[51] Miletic D, Fuckar Z, Sustic A, et al. Resistance and pulsatility indices in acute renal obstruction. J Clin Ultrasound 1998;26:79–84.

[52] Riccabona M, Ring E, Fueger G, et al. Doppler sonography in congenital ureteropelvic junction obstruction and congenital multicystic kidney disease. Pediatr Radiol 1993;23:502–5.

[53] Vade A, Dudiak C, McCarthy P, et al. Resistive indices in the evaluation of infants with obstructive and nonobstructive pyelocaliectasis. J Ultrasound Med 1999;18:357–61.

ULTRASOUND
CLINICS

Ultrasound Clin 1 (2006) 471–483

Sonographic Evaluation of the Child with Lower Abdominal or Pelvic Pain

Peter J. Strouse, MD

- General approach
- Gastrointestinal disorders
- Appendicitis
- Mesenteric adenitis
- Intussusception
- Duplication cyst
- Inflammatory bowel disease
- Henoch-Schönlein purpura
- Meckel diverticulum
- Small bowel obstruction
- Omental infarction
- Urinary tract disorders

  Renal stone
  Urinary tract infection
  Infected urachus
- Gynecologic disorders
  Hematometrocolpos/hematocolpos
  Cyst/ruptured cyst
  Ovarian neoplasms
  Ectopic pregnancy
  Tubo-ovarian abscess
  Ovarian torsion
- Summary
- References

At many centers, CT has become the primary imaging modality for children who have abdominal pain. CT, however, delivers a substantial radiation dose, which is of particular concern in the pediatric patient. In contrast, sonography does not expose the patient to ionizing radiation. Properly performed, sonography is capable of providing useful diagnostic information in the child who has lower abdominal or pelvic pain. In many children and with many disorders, sonography proves to be the only imaging modality that may be required. In this article, the usefulness of sonography in evaluating disorders producing lower abdominal or pelvic pain in a child is reviewed.

General approach

Work-up of the child who has lower abdominal or pelvic pain begins with a careful history and physical examination. Pertinent laboratory examination may be helpful. The decision of whether to image and which modality to use is guided by information obtained from the history, physical examination, and basic laboratory examination.

Abdominal pain is a common complaint in children. It is one of the most common reasons for an unscheduled visit to the pediatrician's office or a visit to an emergency department. The overwhelming majority of children presenting with abdominal pain do not have an organic condition requiring medical or surgical intervention [1,2]. Findings that suggest there is an organic etiology to the patient's complaints of pain are pain that is not periumbilical or pain that migrates from a periumbilical location, fever, leukocytosis, abnormal urinalysis, blood in stool, or a palpable mass. When one of these findings is present, further evaluation with imaging is likely required.

Imaging protocols naturally vary from institution to institution and even between different physician

Section of Pediatric Radiology, C.S. Mott Children's Hospital, Room F3503, Department of Radiology, University of Michigan Health System, 1500 East Medical Center Drive, Ann Arbor, MI 48103-0252, USA
E-mail address: pstrouse@umich.edu

doi:10.1016/j.cult.2006.05.001

users and imaging providers within the same institution. If pathology of the female pelvis is suspected, ultrasound is firmly indicated as an initial imaging step. With suspected gastrointestinal pathology, radiography, sonography, or CT may be used, depending on the suspected disorder, the age of the child, and institutional preferences. This is also true for suspected urinary tract pathology. When there is uncertainty of the origin of a child's pain, preliminary examination with sonography is a good first step, because it does not expose the child to ionizing radiation and it guides the proper use of other imaging studies.

Gastrointestinal disorders

Regardless of the disorder being imaged, evaluation of the gastrointestinal tract with sonography requires meticulous technique. Air is the enemy of the ultrasound beam. Graded compression of the abdomen is required to obliterate and displace gas from bowel in the field of view. Although tensely distended gas filled bowel or guarding by the patient may occasionally obscure visualization, careful, gradual compression usually achieves visualization of deeper structures. Visualization of bowel is improved by use of a linear array transducer. Compression also serves to bring the pathologic bowel in the focal zone ("sweet spot") of the transducer.

Well-trained sonographic technologists may be skilled in performing ultrasound of the gastrointestinal tract; however, the value of witnessing scanning of the patient or, better yet, scanning the patient oneself, cannot be overstated. The realtime capability of sonography allows for a directed scan ("show me where it hurts"). The reaction of the patient to palpation with the transducer also yields information. The suspicion of underlying pathology may be heightened or lessened by observing or performing this limited physical examination.

Appendicitis

Appendicitis is overwhelmingly the most common surgical cause for abdominal pain in childhood. Nonetheless, only a small percentage of children presenting with abdominal pain prove to have appendicitis [1–3]. Clinical findings suggestive of appendicitis include periumbilical pain migrating to the right lower quadrant, fever, and leukocytosis. Until the late 1980s the diagnosis of appendicitis was purely clinical. Unfortunately, clinical evaluation of appendicitis is imprecise. Historically, an accepted 15% to 20% negative appendectomy rate was balanced against a desire to limit complications caused by perforation of undiagnosed appendicitis.

Graded compression ultrasound for the evaluation of appendicitis was introduced by Puylaert in1986 [4]. As previously described, a linear array transducer is used. Compression is applied gradually so as to be better tolerated by the patient. The examination is best started by asking the patient, "Where does it hurt?" (Do *not* tell the patient to "point to where it hurts.") The patient who has uncomplicated appendicitis often points to a specific location. The indicated area of the abdomen is the starting point for scanning. It is striking how often the abnormal appendix is found immediately beneath the site where the patient indicates the pain. If the appendix is not immediately identified, a systematic search of the right lower quadrant and pelvis is performed. Careful sweeps in the longitudinal and transverse planes are performed. Less experienced sonographers frequently make the mistake of not providing adequate compression. With adequate compression, the posterior abdominal wall, the psoas muscle, and the iliac vasculature are seen (Fig. 1). Illustrations in Puylaert's original article nicely demonstrate the degree of compression required [4].

Some investigators have indicated a high rate of identifying the normal appendix [5,6]. To exclude appendicitis, the bulbous tip of the appendix must be seen. Identification of the normal appendix is the best evidence that the patient does not have appendicitis. Identification of the normal appendix, however, is extremely difficult and time consuming.

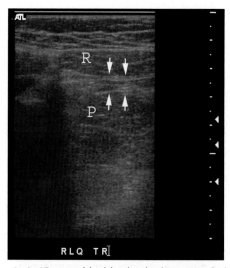

Fig. 1. A 15-year-old girl who had a normal right lower quadrant ultrasound. Adequate compression is indicated by visualization of the posterior abdominal wall, including the psoas muscle (P). Note the short distance (*between the pairs of arrows*) between the rectus abdominus muscle (R) in the anterior abdominal wall and psoas muscle posteriorly.

In most practices and for most patients the normal appendix is never seen. Lack of identification of an abnormal appendix is good evidence against the diagnosis of the appendicitis; however, some uncertainty inevitably persists as to whether an inflamed appendix may have been missed. This uncertainty may be heightened or tempered by witnessing the patient's reaction to being scanned. If the patient is completely comfortable with deep palpation by the transducer, he or she is unlikely to have appendicitis. If the patient is very uncomfortable to minimal compression with the transducer, the likelihood of underlying pathology is higher.

The normal appendix is 6 mm or less in diameter and compressible (Fig. 2). The abnormal appendix is 7 mm or greater in diameter and noncompressible (Fig. 3) [4,5]. The appendix is tubular and blind ending. An appendicolith may or may not be present (Fig. 4). If the appendix is truly abnormal, it should be re-demonstrable—one should be able to verify the abnormality by removing the transducer, replacing it, and re-finding the abnormality. Color Doppler may show increased flow indicating inflammation [7]. In the setting of perforation, the appendix may no longer be visible [8–10]. A mass or abscess may be found [5,8]. Such findings are nonspecific; however, as appendicitis is the most likely diagnosis in this setting, perforated appendicitis should be suspected [9].

In experienced hands, ultrasound performs well in the diagnosis of appendicitis [4,11,12]. Although CT is probably more sensitive and more specific, it is only slightly better than ultrasound. Disadvantages of ultrasound include dependence on the operator and lack of a global view of the abdomen and pelvis [13]. Both of these disadvantages are surmounted by CT. In most head-to-head comparisons, CT exceeds sonography in sensitivity and specificity [13–16]. At most institutions in the United States, CT has thus supplanted ultrasound as the chief diagnostic modality in the diagnosis of appendicitis. This is somewhat unfortunate given the radiation exposure associated with CT and the increasing reliance on imaging for diagnosis, leading to more children with lesser symptoms or suspicion for disease being imaged.

What is the proper role of ultrasound in suspected appendicitis? Before answering this question, it is important to acknowledge that there are two questions asked of us by our surgical colleagues: "Does this child have appendicitis?" And, "Is it perforated?" At many institutions, surgical management of perforated and nonperforated appendicitis differs. In an ideal setting ultrasound serves as a screening examination for appendicitis [12,15,17,18]. Most children who have appendicitis would be diagnosed using sonography, thus avoiding a CT. In cases in which there was a high clinical suspicion or equivocal sonographic findings, CT would be performed. In cases in which perforated appendicitis is strongly suspected, imaging could commence directly with CT. This model has worked well at some pediatric institutions [17,19,20]; however, when one imaging study exceeds another in accuracy (as viewed by our clinical colleagues) it becomes difficult to supplant in clinical work. It is incumbent on radiologists to maintain the skills of appendiceal sonography to provide a radiation-free imaging alternative to CT.

Mesenteric adenitis

The diagnosis of mesenteric adenitis is one of exclusion. This is not a diagnosis that is accepted by all.

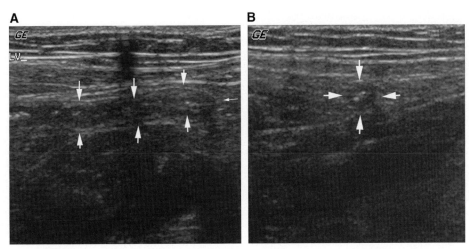

Fig. 2. An 11-year-old girl who had a normal appendix (*arrows*) seen on (*A*) longitudinal and (*B*) transverse views. This appendix is 4 mm in diameter. *Small arrow*, tip of the appendix.

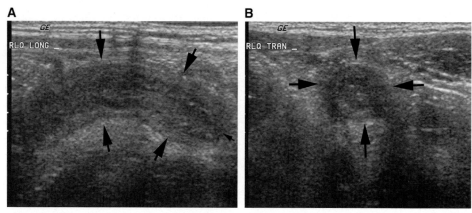

A

GE
RLQ LONG _

B

GE
RLQ TRAN _

Fig. 3. A 5-year-old boy who had nonperforated appendicitis. An enlarged appendix (*arrows*) measuring 12 mm in diameter is seen on (*A*) longitudinal and (*B*) transverse views. *Small arrow*, tip of the appendix.

Children may be assigned the diagnosis of mesenteric adenitis when enlarged lymph nodes are seen in the right lower quadrant in the absence of other pathology (Fig. 5). Mildly prominent right lower quadrant mesenteric lymph nodes are a normal finding in children, and criteria for what constitutes abnormal enlargement are not well defined [21, 22]. Enlarged lymph nodes may also be seen with various pathologies, including appendicitis, inflammatory bowel disease, yersinia ileitis, and Henoch-Schönlein purpura [23]. The diagnosis of mesenteric adenitis is not used at the author's institution.

Intussusception

At many institutions, including the author's, ultrasound has become the chief diagnostic method of confirming the presence of intussusception [24,25]. Improvement of ultrasound equipment has allowed for this development. Concomitantly, an unacceptably high and increasing negative rate for enemas performed for suspected intussusception has prompted the development of new imaging algorithms to avoid numerous unnecessary enema examinations in young children [24,25].

Ultrasound performs well in identifying ileocolic intussusceptions [24–28]. False negatives are rare. Intussusceptions are seen as large masses, usually approximately 4 cm in diameter or greater. The longitudinal dimension of the mass varies depending on the length of the intussusception. Most intussusceptions are encountered in the right midabdomen or subhepatic space; however, the mass can be found anywhere within the abdomen or pelvis. The sonographic search therefore begins in the right midabdomen, but must include the whole abdomen if no intussusception is encountered on the right. In the author's experience, a negative

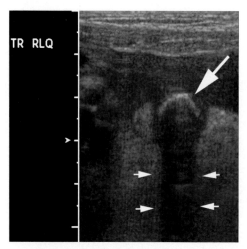

TR RLQ

Fig. 4. A 5-year-old girl who had perforated appendicitis. An appendicolith (*large arrow*) is seen with a posterior acoustic shadow (*small arrows*). A layer of soft tissue around the appendicolith is appendiceal wall. The appendix was not seen otherwise.

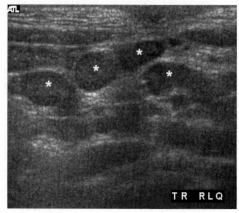

TR RLQ

Fig. 5. A 3-year-old boy who had mildly enlarged right lower quadrant lymph nodes (*asterisks*).

ultrasound is highly predictive of the absence of an intussusception. Rarely, if clinical suspicion persists, an enema still may be performed.

On ultrasound, an ileocolic intussusception is seen as a large mass with a layered appearance or a thick hypoechoic outer wall caused by edematous bowel wall (Fig. 6) [24–29]. The center of the lesion is hyperechoic owing to mesenteric fat within the intussusception. Lymph nodes are often present within the hyperechoic center (Fig. 7) [29,30]. These are seen as small oval hypoechoic structures, usually less than 1 cm. There are no sonographic findings that preclude subsequent enema for treatment; however, some findings have been identified that may indicate a lesser likelihood of successful reduction and a higher likelihood of complicating perforation. These findings include lack of blood flow within the intussusception on Doppler evaluation and trapped fluid within layers on the intussusception [29,31,32].

Other disorders may be mistaken for an ileocolic intussusception. Small bowel intussusceptions appear similar but are smaller in diameter and often transient (Fig. 8) [33]. Disorders that cause bowel wall thickening may appear similar, including inflammatory bowel disease, lymphoma, and intramural hemorrhage.

Ultrasound may also demonstrate findings suggestive of a lead point of an intussusception [34]. Only 5% of pediatric patients have a lead point. Lead points that may be demonstrated by sonography include a duplication cyst or bowel wall thickening caused by inflammation or intramural

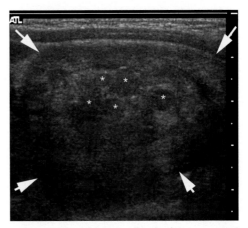

Fig. 7. A 3-year-old boy who had intussusception (*arrows*). Multiple lymph nodes (*asterisks*) are seen within mesenteric fat within the intussusception.

hemorrhage as may be seen with Henoch-Schönlein purpura.

Ultrasound has been used at some institutions to monitor reduction of intussusception with saline, water, and even air enemas [35,36]. This further spares the patient radiation exposure. A disadvantage of the technique is a limited field of view during the reduction. This technique has had very limited use in the United States.

Duplication cyst

Classic duplication cysts have a characteristic appearance on ultrasound of the double layered wall (Fig. 9) [37,38]. The inner layer is hyperechoic mucosa and the outer layer is hypoechoic muscle. Unfortunately with inflammation, the layers may be

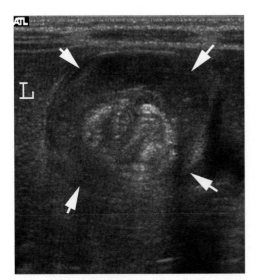

Fig. 6. A 4-month-old boy who had intussusception (*arrows*). A thick hypoechoic "donut" is seen with echogenic mesenteric fat centrally within the mass. L, liver.

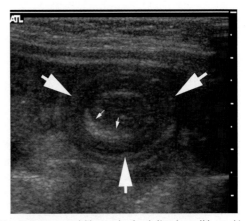

Fig. 8. A 3-year-old boy who had distal small bowel intussusception caused by Henoch-Schönlein purpura. The intussusception (*large arrows*) is less than 2 cm in diameter, much smaller than the typical ileocolic intussusception. *Small arrows*, mesenteric fat within the intussusception.

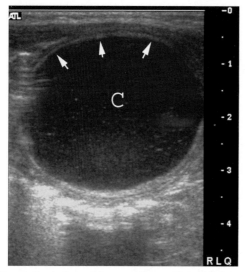

Fig. 9. An infant girl presenting with small bowel obstruction secondary to volvulus around an enteric duplication cyst. This cyst (C) measures 3.5 cm in diameter. Portions of the cyst wall show the characteristic double-layered appearance with echogenic mucosa internally (*arrows*) and hypoechoic muscle externally.

obscured, lessening the specificity [39]. Nonetheless, demonstration of a cystic mass adjacent to bowel should prompt consideration of a duplication cyst.

Duplication cysts are congenital malformations of bowel that can occur anywhere in the gastrointestinal tract [38,40]. The most common locations are at the esophagus followed by terminal ileum [40]. Classically, children present early in childhood as the cyst distends with fluid. If gastric mucosa is present within the cyst, it may secrete enzymes, leading to inflammation and presentation with pain.

Differential considerations for a fluid-filled cystic mass in the lower abdomen include omental or mesenteric cysts and ovarian neoplasm. Omental and mesenteric cysts are usually asymptomatic unto themselves, unless there is an associated obstruction or torsion of bowel.

Inflammatory bowel disease

Inflammatory bowel disease produces bowel wall thickening [41]. If a segment of small bowel or colon with a thick wall is identified by sonography, the diagnosis should be suspected. Differentiation of abnormal small bowel from abnormal colon may be difficult, but may be inferred by anatomic location. Correlation with clinical presentation is helpful. The inflamed small bowel of Crohn disease is typically on the order of 3 cm in diameter, substantially larger than the typical inflamed appendix. In transverse, the appearance is similar to an intussusception; however, in longitudinal views the abnormal bowel is more elongate and does not have the overlapped or invaginated appearance of an intussusception (Fig. 10). Hyperemia is evident on Doppler interrogation. Occasionally hypertrophied adipose tissue is seen adjacent to the inflamed loop of bowel. This tissue appears homogeneously hyperechoic.

At some centers, mostly in Europe, sonography has been used to longitudinally monitor Crohn disease activity [41,42].

Other infectious or inflammatory bowel diseases may appear similar to Crohn disease, including

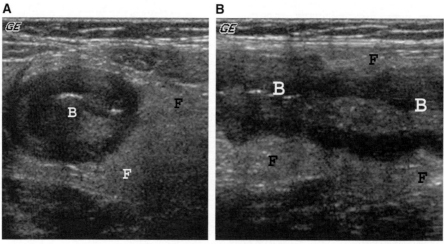

Fig. 10. A 9-year-old girl who had acute abdominal pain as the presenting manifestation of Crohn disease. (*A*) Transverse and (*B*) longitudinal images show an abnormal segment of small bowel (B) with prominent echogenic mucosa centrally and a markedly thickened wall. Note prominent adjacent fat (F).

ulcerative colitis, pseudomembranous colitis, yersinia ileitis, and infectious entero-colitides. In a neutropenic patient, marked thickening of the cecal and proximal ascending colon wall may indicate typhlitis (neutropenic colitis). Correlation with clinical history and physical examination may help differentiate inflammatory disorders causing bowel wall thickening.

Henoch-Schönlein purpura

Henoch-Schönlein purpura (HSP) is an idiopathic vasculitis. Although the disorder may involve several organ systems, the chief sources of morbidity are involvement of the gastrointestinal and genitourinary tract [43]. These children develop a characteristic purpuric rash; however, involvement of the gastrointestinal tract may precede development of the rash.

In children who have HSP, the bowel wall is thickened by inflammation and intramural hemorrhage (Fig. 11) [43–45]. Bowel wall abnormality is often discontinuous. Increased flow is seen on Doppler interrogation. Free intraperitoneal fluid and mild mesenteric lymph node enlargement are common findings. The mural abnormality of HSP may act as a lead point for an intussusception (see Fig. 8) [43,44]. If the patient has not yet been diagnosed with HSP, the finding of bowel wall thickening, with or without an intussusception, should prompt consideration of the diagnosis.

Meckel diverticulum

Meckel diverticulum is a remnant of the omphalomesenteric duct [46]. Meckel diverticulum can present in various ways. In addition to the classic presentation with painless gastrointestinal hemorrhage, Meckel diverticulum can present with inflammation (Meckel diverticulitis), as a lead point for an intussusception, or as the focal point of a small bowel volvulus (usually in association with an omphalomesenteric band) [26,46].

Meckel diverticulum is rarely diagnosed prospectively; however, sonography may identify the inflamed diverticulum, an intussusception, or a small bowel obstruction caused by a Meckel diverticulum [26,46]. Identification of the appendix as separate from the area of inflammation, location to the left of midline, and larger size than is typical for an inflamed appendix all suggest Meckel diverticulitis as opposed to appendicitis [46,47].

Small bowel obstruction

Children who have small bowel obstruction are often evaluated with means other than ultrasound, because the history and physical examination findings lead the clinician to suspect the presence of an obstruction. Many of the previously discussed entities may cause a small bowel obstruction. The presence of fluid-filled dilated loops on sonography may suggest an obstruction, particularly if a caliber change is demonstrated and collapsed loops are seen further distal. Sonography may be helpful in demonstrating the cause of an obstruction (Fig. 12) [48].

Omental infarction

Omental infarction is usually caused by torsion of an omental appendage. The cause for torsion and infarction is unknown. In some patients the onset of symptoms has been linked to a large meal. Patients present with sudden onset pain. Patients are usually but not invariably afebrile and without elevation of the white blood cell count. The clinical presentation may mimic appendicitis.

Although the diagnosis is more readily made by CT, sonography can also make the diagnosis, particularly when the operator is familiar with the entity and searches for the findings. On ultrasound, the infarcted omentum is seen as a lenticular or ovoid mass immediately behind the anterior abdominal wall, usually in the right lower quadrant [49,50]. The mass is homogeneous and hyperechoic and corresponds with the patient's point of maximal tenderness.

Omental infarction is a self-limited condition. Surgery is not required. Making the diagnosis may spare the patient an unnecessary surgery.

Urinary tract disorders

Renal stone

Renal colic is in the differential diagnosis for lower abdominal pain in children. Pain is usually referred to the flank, but may present in the lower abdomen or pelvis. Renal calculi are much less common in children than in adults; however, they are not infrequently encountered [51]. Use of CT for the diagnosis of renal calculi has become commonplace even in children; however, the radiation dose associated with CT must be considered [52]. At initial presentation with a calculus, the diagnosis may not initially be entertained and ultrasound may be performed. In a child who has a history of calculi, performance of repeated renal stone protocol CT studies is to be discouraged, particularly if the clinical presentation is consistent with a recurrent calculus. Ultrasound can be useful in these children to evaluate for collecting system dilatation, which together with the clinical presentation offers confirmatory evidence of the presence of an obstructing

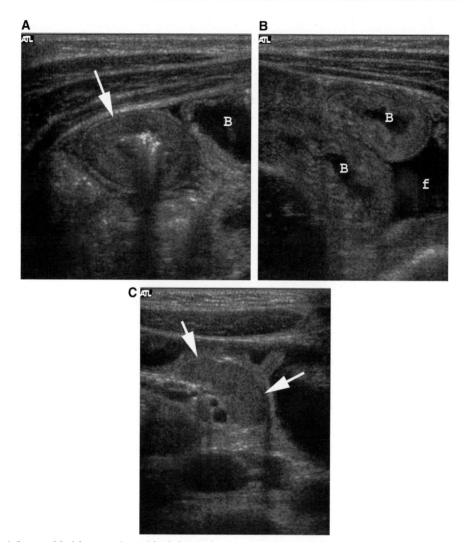

Fig. 11. A 6-year-old girl presenting with abdominal pain caused by Henoch-Schönlein purpura. (A) An involved bowel loop (arrow) with a thick wall is seen adjacent to a normal bowel loop (B). (B) Additional thick-walled bowel loops seen in longitudinal view. F, free fluid. (C) Mildly enlarged lymph nodes (arrows).

calculus [53]. Occasionally sonography may demonstrate an impacted distal ureteral calculus (Fig. 13).

Urinary tract infection

Children who have cystitis caused by lower urinary tract infection or other causes may present with pelvic pain. Sonography may show thickening of the urinary bladder wall. Unfortunately, thickening of the bladder wall is difficult to interpret. The wall of an underdistended bladder may appear very thick. Thickening disproportionate to the degree of distension, irregularity, and asymmetry of thickening are features that suggest pathologic bladder wall thickening as opposed to spurious thickening from underdistention.

Upper urinary tract infections usually present flank pain higher in the abdomen, as do other disorders of the kidney.

Infected urachus

Infected urachus is a rare cause of lower abdominal pain. The urachus is an embryonic connection from the anterior aspect of the dome of the bladder to the umbilicus [54]. The urachus may persist in its entirety (patent urachus) or either end (urachal sinus, urachal diverticulum). If the midportion persists with both ends obliterated, the patient may develop a urachal cyst. These cysts are often asymptomatic until they become superinfected. On sonography, a complex, cystic mass is identified at the midline

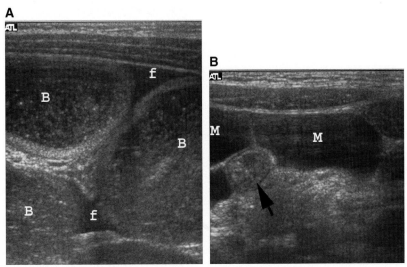

Fig. 12. A 3-year-old boy who had small bowel obstruction caused by focal volvulus related to a mesenteric cyst. (*A*) Dilated small bowel loops (B) containing fecal material, consistent with a small bowel obstruction. F, free fluid. (*B*) The mesenteric cyst (M) is seen as a septated, fluid-filled mass. Note that it partially encases a normal caliber bowel loop (*arrow*).

between umbilicus and bladder [54], and there may be surrounding inflammation.

Gynecologic disorders

Hematometrocolpos/hematocolpos

Hematometrocolpos presenting in adolescent girls is usually secondary to vaginal obstruction by an imperforate hymen. The patient presents at puberty with primary amenorrhea and cyclic lower abdominal or pelvic pain. Ultrasound shows a fluid-filled mass posterior to the bladder representing the dilated vagina. The uterus may (hematometrocolpos) or may not (hematocolpos) be dilated also. The dilated uterus can be differentiated from the vagina by the cervical margin and thicker wall. Occasionally the fallopian tubes may be dilated.

Hematometros and hematometrocolpos may also occur because of congenital uterine and vaginal anomalies presenting at the time of puberty, caused by obstruction and distension in response to the onset of menses [55]. Not infrequently in such patients, a duplication is present with obstruction of one side.

Cyst/ruptured cyst

A ruptured functional cyst or corpus luteum cyst is a common cause of pelvic pain in teenage girls [56]. Usually the causal cyst is no longer evident because it has decompressed itself through rupture. Sometimes a hyperechoic or complex cystic mass of the ovary persists. A variable amount of free fluid is present within the pelvis. Debris from hemorrhage may be present within the fluid.

Ovarian or paraovarian cysts may cause pain in themselves. Ovarian cysts in adolescent girls are usually functional cysts, forming in response to the cycling hormones of the menstrual cycle. Given the low incidence of malignant ovarian tumors, it is usually sufficient to obtain a follow-up sonogram after at least one full menstrual cycle to confirm resolution of the finding.

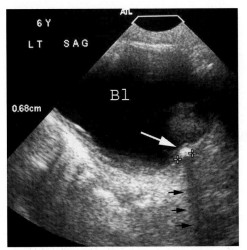

Fig. 13. A 6-year-old girl who had impacted distal ureteral calculus (*large arrow*). A posterior acoustic shadow (*small arrows*) is seen. Bl, bladder.

Ovarian neoplasms

Ovarian neoplasms in children are usually benign [57,58]. Most tumors present as a painless mass;

however, some tumors present with pelvic pain, particularly if the tumor is acting as a nidus for torsion. As discussed previously, functional cysts are the most common cause of an ovarian mass [56,57]. Persistence of the cyst on follow-up examination, continued symptoms, or identification of any solid component within the mass are all features that may suggest neoplasm.

Ectopic pregnancy

In the sexually active teenage girl, ectopic pregnancy is an important consideration in the differential diagnosis of pelvic pain [59]. Ectopic pregnancy can be life threatening because of hemorrhage. If a patient who has pelvic pain has been sexually active, a pregnancy test is warranted. If the pregnancy test is positive and no intrauterine pregnancy is found, ectopic pregnancy must be strongly considered until proven otherwise. The differential diagnosis for a positive pregnancy test without demonstration of an intrauterine gestation is early intrauterine pregnancy, spontaneous abortion, or ectopic pregnancy. Serial serum β-HCG levels and serial sonography may help to differentiate these possibilities.

Sonography may demonstrate a living ectopic pregnancy outside of the uterus. A gestational sac may be seen in the adnexa (Fig. 14). Findings of adnexal mass and free fluid are nonspecific, but in the setting of a positive pregnancy test and lack of a demonstrable intrauterine pregnancy, these findings are suggestive of an ectopic pregnancy [60,61]. Endovaginal scanning is preferred when evaluating for early pregnancy and possible ectopic pregnancy [62].

Tubo-ovarian abscess

Unfortunately pelvic inflammatory disease and tubo-ovarian abscess are also not infrequent diagnoses in the sexually active teenager [63,64]. In a sexually active teenage girl, gynecologic infection should be in the differential diagnosis for lower abdominal or pelvic pain. A good history and physical examination, including a pelvic examination, may suggest the correct diagnosis. The clinical presentation and physical examination findings overlap with appendicitis, particularly when the pathology is on the right. Sonography is the study of choice in these patients. It demonstrates abnormalities related to the gynecologic tract, and graded compression examination of the right lower quadrant can be performed during the same examination to assess for appendicitis.

In the absence of tubal obstruction, sonographic findings with pelvic inflammatory disease may be normal. Pelvic inflammation may blur margins of the uterus. Free fluid may be present but is nonspecific. Fluid-filled adnexal tubular structures or complex cystic masses in the presence of clinical findings suggesting infection should raise concern for tubo-ovarian abscess (Fig. 15) [64].

Ovarian torsion

Ovarian torsion may occur in a child of any age, but is most common in the neonate and in the adolescent. Increased incidence of ovarian torsion in neonates may relate to enlargement of the ovaries related to stimulation from maternal hormones. The incidence increases again at adolescence in response to hormonal changes. Although underlying masses may act as a nidus for torsion and do

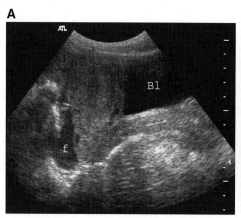
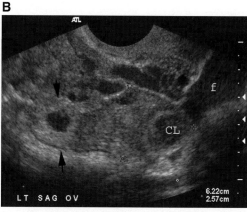

Fig. 14. A teenage girl who had an ectopic pregnancy. The patient was 9 weeks from her last period, had a β-HCG level of 3370 mIU/mL, and presented with acute left pelvic pain. (*A*) Transabdominal images show an empty uterine cavity and free fluid (F). Cursors delimit the uterus. Bl, bladder. Absence of intrauterine pregnancy was confirmed by endovaginal scanning. (*B*) Endovaginal image of the left adnexa. An ectopic tubal ring (*arrows*) is identified adjacent to the left ovary (*cursors*). A corpus luteum is seen within the ovary (CL). F, free fluid. (Images courtesy of Alexis V. Nees, MD, Ann Arbor, Michigan).

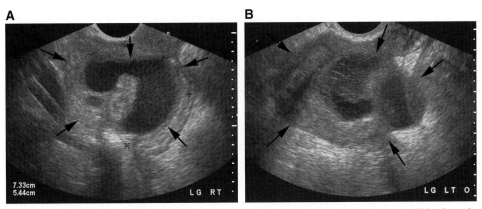

Fig. 15. A teenage girl who had bilateral tubo-ovarian abscesses. Complex, cystic, and solid adnexal masses (*arrows*) are seen on the (*A*) right and (*B*) left. (Images courtesy of Alexis V. Nees, MD, Ann Arbor, Michigan).

increase the risk for torsion, most torsed ovaries in children do not bear an underlying lesion. It is believed that abnormal fixation of the ovary may predispose these ovaries to torsion.

Patients who have ovarian torsion present with sudden onset pelvic or lower abdominal pain. There is often a history of similar episodes of pain before presentation. The patient may have a slight fever and borderline elevation of the white blood cell count, often confounding the clinical diagnosis. On physical examination, a tender mass may be felt.

If there is an underlying mass, it is well shown by sonography. A torsed ovary with a cyst may mimic a gastrointestinal duplication in appearance, occasionally showing a double-layered wall [65]. In torsed ovaries without an underlying mass, the ovary itself appears as a mass because of swelling. The sonographic appearance of the torsed ovary varies from completely solid to cystic, with most having a predominantly solid or mixed solid and cystic appearance [66,67]. The only gray scale finding considered specific for ovarian torsion is a solid mass with small cysts (follicles) at its periphery (Fig. 16). The torsed ovary usually sits in the cul de sac behind the uterus or unusually anterior. Normal ovary is not seen at the expected adnexal location. The value of Doppler interrogation of the torsed ovary is somewhat limited [67]. In the prepubertal ovary, flow may be difficult to demonstrate in a normal ovary, making it difficult to determine if flow is absent. The ovary has dual blood supply from the ovarian and uterine arteries. Flow thus may be present even in the presence of torsion. Nonetheless, if flow is not demonstrable within an enlarged ovary and flow is demonstrable within the contralateral normal ovary, torsion should be suspected.

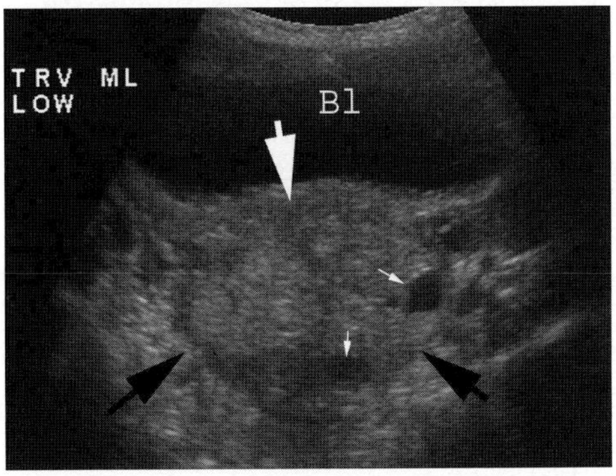

The CT findings of torsion are less specific; however, CT may also demonstrate peripheral follicles within a torsed ovary. Sonography may be helpful in confirming the diagnosis when CT findings are equivocal.

Summary

Sonography is an excellent modality for the evaluation of the child who has lower abdominal or pelvic pain. Whether or not a specific diagnosis (ie, appendicitis) is suspected, versatility and lack of ionizing radiation make sonography an excellent first line of imaging.

References

[1] Buchert GS. Abdominal pain in children: an emergency practitioner's guide. Emerg Med Clin North Am 1989;7:497–517.

[2] Scholer SJ, Pituch K, Orr DP, et al. Clinical outcomes of children with acute abdominal pain. Pediatrics 1996;98:680–5.

[3] Reynolds SL, Jaffe DM. Diagnosing abdominal pain in a pediatric emergency department. Pediatr Emerg Care 1992;8:126–8.

[4] Puylaert JB. Acute appendicitis: US evaluation using graded compression. Radiology 1986; 158:355–60.

Fig. 16. A 2-year-old girl who had a torsed ovary (*large arrows*). A solid mass is seen posterior to the bladder (Bl). Note some peripheral follicles (*small arrows*).

[5] Sivit CJ. Diagnosis of acute appendicitis in children: spectrum of sonographic findings. Am J Roentgenol 1993;161:147–52.

[6] Wiersma F, Sramek A, Holscher HC. US features of the normal appendix and surrounding area in children. Radiology 2005;235:1018–22.

[7] Quillin SP, Siegel MJ. Appendicitis: efficacy of color Doppler sonography. Radiology 1994;191:557–60.

[8] Quillin SP, Siegel MJ, Coffin CM. Acute appendicitis in children: value of sonography in detecting perforation. Am J Roentgenol 1992;159:1265–8.

[9] Borushok KF, Jeffrey RB Jr, Laing FC, et al. Sonographic diagnosis of perforation in patients with acute appendicitis. Am J Roentgenol 1990;154:275–8.

[10] Hayden CK Jr, Kuchelmeister J, Lipscomb TS. Sonography of acute appendicitis in childhood: perforation versus nonperforation. J Ultrasound Med 1992;11:209–16.

[11] Hahn HB, Hoepner FU, Kalle T, et al. Sonography of acute appendicitis in children: 7 years experience. Pediatr Radiol 1998;28:147–51.

[12] Dilley A, Wesson D, Munden M, et al. The impact of ultrasound examinations on the management of children with suspected appendicitis: a 3-year analysis. J Pediatr Surg 2001;36:303–8.

[13] Sivit CJ. Controversies in emergency radiology: acute appendicitis in children—the case for CT. Emerg Radiol 2004;10:238–40.

[14] Applegate KE, Sivit CJ, Salvator AE, et al. Effect of cross-sectional imaging on negative appendectomy and perforation rates in children. Radiology 2001;220:103–7.

[15] Kaiser S, Frenckner B, Jorulf HK. Suspected appendicitis in children: US and CT—a prospective randomized study. Radiology 2002;223:633–8.

[16] Sivit CJ, Applegate KE, Stallion A, et al. Imaging evaluation of suspected appendicitis in a pediatric population: effectiveness of sonography versus CT. Am J Roentgenol 2000;175:977–80.

[17] Garcia Pena BM, Taylor GA, Fishman SJ, et al. Effect of an imaging protocol on clinical outcomes among pediatric patients with appendicitis. Pediatrics 2002;110:1088–93.

[18] Puig S, Hörmann M, Rebhandl W, et al. US as a primary diagnostic tool in relation to negative appendectomy: six years experience. Radiology 2003;226:101–4.

[19] Garcia Pena BM, Taylor GA, Fishman SJ, et al. Costs and effectiveness of ultrasonography and limited computed tomography for diagnosing appendicitis in children. Pediatrics 2000;106:672–6.

[20] Garcia Pena BM, Mandl KD, Kraus SJ, et al. Ultrasonography and limited computed tomography in the diagnosis and management of appendicitis in children. JAMA 1999;282:1041–6.

[21] Vayner N, Coret A, Polliack G, et al. Mesenteric lymphadenopathy in children examined by US for chronic and/or recurrent abdominal pain. Pediatr Radiol 2003;33:864–7.

[22] Karmazyn B, Werner EA, Rejaie B, et al. Mesenteric lymph nodes in children: what is normal? Pediatr Radiol 2005;35:774–7.

[23] Puylaert JB. Mesenteric adenitis and acute terminal ileitis: US evaluation using graded compression. Radiology 1986;161:691–5.

[24] Eshed I, Gorenstein A, Serour F, et al. Intussusception in children: can we rely on screening sonography performed by junior residents? Pediatr Radiol 2004;34:134–7.

[25] Henrikson S, Blane CE, Koujok K, et al. The effect of screening sonography on the positive rate of enemas for intussusception. Pediatr Radiol 2003;33:190–3.

[26] Daneman A, Navarro O. Intussusception. Part 1: a review of diagnostic approaches. Pediatr Radiol 2003;33:79–85.

[27] Shanbhogue RL, Hussain SM, Meradji M, et al. Ultrasonography is accurate enough for the diagnosis of intussusception. J Pediatr Surg 1994;29:324–7 [discussion 327–8].

[28] Verschelden P, Filiatrault D, Garel L, et al. Intussusception in children: reliability of US in diagnosis—a prospective study. Radiology 1992;184:741–4.

[29] del-Pozo G, Albillos JC, Tejedor D. Intussusception: US findings with pathologic correlation—the crescent-in-doughnut sign. Radiology 1996;199:688–92.

[30] Koumanidou C, Vakaki M, Pitsoulakis G, et al. Sonographic detection of lymph nodes in the intussusception of infants and young children: clinical evaluation and hydrostatic reduction. Am J Roentgenol 2002;178:445–50.

[31] del-Pozo G, Gonzalez-Spinola J, Gomez-Anson B, et al. Intussusception: trapped peritoneal fluid detected with US—relationship to reducibility and ischemia. Radiology 1996;201:379–83.

[32] Lim HK, Bae SH, Lee KH, et al. Assessment of reducibility of ileocolic intussusception in children: usefulness of color Doppler sonography. Radiology 1994;191:781–5.

[33] Kim JH. US features of transient small bowel intussusception in pediatric patients. Korean J Radiol 2004;5:178–84.

[34] Navarro O, Daneman A. Intussusception. Part 3: diagnosis and management of those with an identifiable or predisposing cause and those that reduce spontaneously. Pediatr Radiol 2004;34:305–12. quiz 369.

[35] Woo SK, Kim JS, Suh SJ, et al. Childhood intussusception: US-guided hydrostatic reduction. Radiology 1992;182:77–80.

[36] Yoon CH, Kim HJ, Goo HW. Intussusception in children: US-guided pneumatic reduction—initial experience. Radiology 2001;218:85–8.

[37] Teele RL, Henschke CI, Tapper D. The radiographic and ultrasonographic evaluation of enteric duplication cysts. Pediatr Radiol 1980;10:9–14.

[38] Macpherson RI. Gastrointestinal tract duplications: clinical, pathologic, etiologic, and radiologic considerations. Radiographics 1993;13:1063–80.

[39] Cheng G, Soboleski D, Daneman A, et al. Sonographic pitfalls in the diagnosis of enteric duplication cysts. Am J Roentgenol 2005;184:521–5.

[40] Bower RJ, Sieber WK, Kiesewetter WB. Alimentary tract duplications in children. Ann Surg 1978;188:669–74.

[41] Faure C, Belarbi N, Mougenot JF, et al. Ultrasonographic assessment of inflammatory bowel disease in children: comparison with ileocolonoscopy. J Pediatr 1997;130:147–51.

[42] Haber HP, Busch A, Ziebach R, et al. Bowel wall thickness measured by ultrasound as a marker of Crohn's disease activity in children. Lancet 2000; 355:1239–40.

[43] Chang WL, Yang YH, Lin YT, et al. Gastrointestinal manifestations in Henoch-Schönlein purpura: a review of 261 patients. Acta Paediatr 2004;93:1427–31.

[44] Bomelburg T, Claasen U, von Lengerke HJ. Intestinal ultrasonographic findings in Schönlein-Henoch syndrome. Eur J Pediatr 1991;150:158–60.

[45] Ozdemir H, Isik S, Buyan N, et al. Sonographic demonstration of intestinal involvement in Henoch-Schönlein syndrome. Eur J Radiol 1995; 20:32–4.

[46] Levy AD, Hobbs CM. From the archives of the AFIP. Meckel diverticulum: radiologic features with pathologic correlation. Radiographics 2004;24:565–87.

[47] Baldisserotto M, Maffazzoni DR, Dora MD. Sonographic findings of Meckel's diverticulitis in children. Am J Roentgenol 2003;180:425–8.

[48] Traubici J, Daneman A, Wales P, et al. Mesenteric lymphatic malformation associated with small-bowel volvulus—two cases and a review of the literature. Pediatr Radiol 2002;32:362–5.

[49] Baldisserotto M, Maffazzoni DR, Dora MD. Omental infarction in children: color Doppler sonography correlated with surgery and pathology findings. Am J Roentgenol 2005;184:156–62.

[50] Grattan-Smith JD, Blews DE, Brand T. Omental infarction in pediatric patients: sonographic and CT findings. Am J Roentgenol 2002;178: 1537–9.

[51] Nimkin K, Lebowitz RL, Share JC, et al. Urolithiasis in a children's hospital: 1985–1990. Urol Radiol 1992;14:139–43.

[52] Strouse PJ, Bates DG, Bloom DA, et al. Noncontrast thin-section helical CT of urinary tract calculi in children. Pediatr Radiol 2002; 32:326–32.

[53] Smith SL, Somers JM, Broderick N, et al. The role of the plain radiograph and renal tract ultrasound in the management of children with renal tract calculi. Clin Radiol 2000;55:708–10.

[54] Yu JS, Kim KW, Lee HJ, et al. Urachal remnant diseases: spectrum of CT and US findings. Radiographics 2001;21:451–61.

[55] Blask AR, Sanders RC, Rock JA. Obstructed uterovaginal anomalies: demonstration with sonography. Part II. Teenagers. Radiology 1991; 179:84–8.

[56] Baltarowich OH, Kurtz AB, Pasto ME, et al. The spectrum of sonographic findings in hemorrhagic ovarian cysts. Am J Roentgenol 1987; 148:901–5.

[57] de Silva KS, Kanumakala S, Grover SR, et al. Ovarian lesions in children and adolescents—an 11-year review. J Pediatr Endocrinol Metab 2004; 17:951–7.

[58] Surratt JT, Siegel MJ. Imaging of pediatric ovarian masses. Radiographics 1991;11:533–48.

[59] Ammerman S, Shafer MA, Snyder D. Ectopic pregnancy in adolescents: a clinical review for pediatricians. J Pediatr 1990;117:677–86.

[60] Dialani V, Levine D. Ectopic pregnancy: a review. Ultrasound Q 2004;20:105–17.

[61] Frates MC, Laing FC. Sonographic evaluation of ectopic pregnancy: an update. Am J Roentgenol 1995;165:251–9.

[62] Bellah RD, Rosenberg HK. Transvaginal ultrasound in a children's hospital: is it worthwhile? Pediatr Radiol 1991;21:570–4.

[63] Banikarim C, Chacko MR. Pelvic inflammatory disease in adolescents. Adolesc Med Clin 2004; 15:273–85. [viii.].

[64] Bulas DI, Ahlstrom PA, Sivit CJ, et al. Pelvic inflammatory disease in the adolescent: comparison of transabdominal and transvaginal sonographic evaluation. Radiology 1992;183: 435–9.

[65] Godfrey H, Abernethy L, Boothroyd A. Torsion of an ovarian cyst mimicking enteric duplication cyst on transabdominal ultrasound: two cases. Pediatr Radiol 1998;28:171–3.

[66] Graif M, Itzchak Y. Sonographic evaluation of ovarian torsion in childhood and adolescence. Am J Roentgenol 1988;150:647–9.

[67] Stark JE, Siegel MJ. Ovarian torsion in prepubertal and pubertal girls: sonographic findings. Am J Roentgenol 1994;163:1479–82.

ELSEVIER
SAUNDERS

U L T R A S O U N D
C L I N I C S

Ultrasound Clin 1 (2006) 485–496

The Acute Pediatric Scrotum

Brian D. Coley, MD[a,b,]*

- Testicular torsion
  Intravaginal torsion
  Extravaginal torsion
- Appendiceal torsion
- Epididymitis and orchitis
  Acute epididymitis
  Orchitis
- Trauma

- Varicocele
- Inguinal hernia
- Hydrocele
- Idiopathic scrotal edema
- Henoch-Schönlein purpura
- Summary
- References

The acute scrotum is defined as the sudden onset of scrotal pain, often accompanied by swelling and redness or discoloration. The differential diagnostic possibilities for the acute scrotum depend on the patient's age. In the neonate the principle diagnoses are testicular torsion (pre- or postnatal), meconium peritonitis/orchitis, hernias, and hydroceles. In the older child, principal diagnoses include testicular torsion, appendage testis, or epididymis torsion, and epididymitis. Less common entities include trauma, hernias and hydroceles, vasculitis, peritonitis, and idiopathic scrotal edema. Testicular torsion is always the primary concern, because testicular salvage is directly related to duration of torsion. Testicular torsion requires immediate surgical intervention, whereas most other causes of acute scrotal pain can be managed medically.

Although the rapidity of symptom onset, associated symptoms, and physical examination findings may suggest the diagnosis [1], imaging is often required. Ultrasound with color Doppler is the imaging modality of choice for scrotal evaluation and has proven to be highly sensitive and specific in the diagnosis of acute scrotal pain [2,3].

Testicular torsion

Intravaginal torsion

Testicular torsion (also referred to as spermatic cord torsion) has two incidence peaks, one in the perinatal period and one around puberty. In the peripubertal period, testicular torsion is intravaginal, with the testis and spermatic cord twisting within the tunica vaginalis caused by improper fixation of the testis (bell-clapper deformity). The twisting of the spermatic cord results first in compromised venous outflow and ultimately arterial inflow, leading to testicular ischemia and eventual infarction. Among children and adolescents presenting with acute scrotal pain, spermatic cord torsion is present in 6% to 31% [2,4–8]. Of all the causes of acute scrotal pain, the onset of symptoms is most rapid for testicular torsion. Nausea and vomiting are more common in testicular torsion and have a positive predictive value of more than 96% [9,10]. Physical examination findings include swelling, an abnormal transverse lie of the testis within the scrotum, and loss of the cremasteric reflex. The physical examination may be difficult to perform in an ill

[a] Department of Radiology, Columbus Children's Hospital, Columbus, OH, USA
[b] Department of Radiology and Pediatrics, The Ohio State University College of Medicine and Public Health, Columbus, OH, USA
* Department of Radiology, Columbus Children's Hospital, 700 Children's Drive, Columbus, OH 43205, USA
E-mail address: bcoley@chi.osu.edu

doi:10.1016/j.cult.2006.05.002

child, however, and histories are not always clear. If the history and physical examination strongly suggest torsion, the patient should go directly to surgery without any delay to perform imaging studies [1]. Imaging should be used for those patients who have unclear diagnoses, in whom torsion is unlikely and another diagnosis needs to be addressed, and in those who have symptoms lasting longer than 24 hours, because even if torsion is present, the chance of testicular salvage is remote and emergency surgery may not be required.

The treatment for testicular torsion is emergent surgery with detorsion and fixation of the testis to the scrotal wall, along with contralateral orchidopexy, because the bell-clapper deformity is often bilateral. Manual detorsion can be performed to minimize ischemia while waiting for surgery and has been reported to have good success [11]. Testicular survival is directly related to the time from onset of symptoms, with only 20% salvage after 12 hours and virtually no salvage after 24 hours. Nonviable testes are removed to prevent immune-mediated injury to the contralateral testis [12,13].

Early sonographic literature focused on changes in parenchymal echotexture caused by ischemia, which were of limited value. In general, the acutely torsed testis is more hypoechoic than normal. The gray-scale findings in testicular torsion, however, are seldom normal. Useful gray-scale findings for torsion include an abnormal transverse testicular lie and a paratesticular "mass" composed of swollen edematous epididymis and spermatic cord [14] (Fig. 1). In some cases, the actual twist of the spermatic cord can be visualized [15–18] (Fig. 2). A reactive hydrocele and scrotal skin thickening is often present, particularly in later cases. If there is

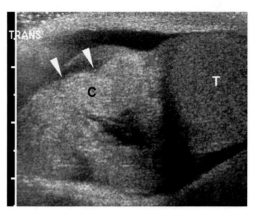

Fig. 2. Testicular torsion. Transverse sonogram shows an echogenic spermatic cord (C) with undulating indentations (*arrowheads*) indicating cord twisting. T, testis.

surrounding fluid, the presence of the bell-clapper deformity is sometimes demonstrated by showing lack of fixation of the testicle to the scrotal wall. As ischemia and infarction progress, the testis becomes heterogeneous, which portends nonviability [19].

To diagnose testicular torsion, one must definitively demonstrate reduced or absent blood flow to the symptomatic testis and normal blood flow to the asymptomatic testis. The sensitivity of color Doppler examination with newer ultrasound equipment in detecting acute testicular torsion in children is 90% to 100%, with the specificity of technically adequate studies being essentially 100% [3]. Although there have been studies examining alterations in venous waveforms, the hallmark of testicular torsion is absent or diminished arterial flow relative to the asymptomatic contralateral testis (Fig. 3). The presence of flow in the painful testis does not exclude the diagnosis of torsion. Color Doppler should be used to perform a semiquantitative estimate of blood flow symmetry. Early or partial cord torsion is not uncommon [20–23], and these testes may demonstrate arterial flow, albeit diminished in quantity from the asymptomatic contralateral testis and with diminished diastolic flow [24,25] (Fig. 4).

A nonsurgical painful testis must be hyperemic relative to the asymptomatic side, otherwise torsion remains a diagnostic possibility. Exceptions to this are cases of spontaneous detorsion, which results in increased blood flow to the testis and peritesticular tissues, giving the appearance of an inflammatory nonsurgical condition [20,21,26,27] (Fig. 5). Spontaneous detorsion is usually accompanied by a marked relief in symptoms, however, which can help clarify the situation. Although spontaneous detorsion is not a surgical emergency, affected

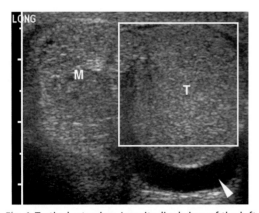

Fig. 1. Testicular torsion. Longitudinal view of the left scrotum shows an abnormal position of the testis (T), which is imaged in transverse section. No flow was demonstrable. There is a large paratesticular mass (M) composed of epididymis and cord tissues and a reactive hydrocele (*arrowhead*).

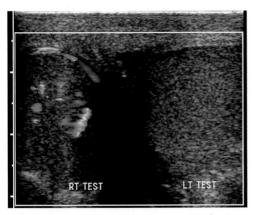

Fig. 3. Acute testicular torsion. Transverse color Doppler sonogram shows blood flow to the normal right testis, but no flow to the symptomatic left testis, indicating torsion.

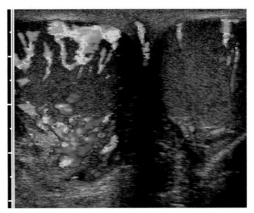

Fig. 5. Detorsion. Transverse color Doppler sonogram of the testes after detorsion of a painful right testis shows marked hyperemia of the right testis. The patient was nearly pain free at the time of the ultrasound and underwent operative fixation the next morning.

patients are at risk for subsequent torsion and should undergo orchidopexy [11,21].

The sonographic findings in late torsion (greater than 24 hours) become more dramatic, with the testicle often becoming disorganized and heterogeneous because of infarction. Peritesticular soft tissue inflammation becomes marked. Color Doppler shows hyperemia of the scrotum and peritesticular tissues with absent flow to the testis (Fig. 6), corresponding to the "doughnut sign" seen with scintigraphy. If not removed, the infarcted testis begins to atrophy, often becoming hyperechoic because of fibrosis or calcification [3]. Changes in the epididymis are also common, as are hydroceles.

Extravaginal torsion

Extravaginal torsion occurs in neonates because of poor fixation of the spermatic cord within the

inguinal canal, allowing the entire cord to twist and compromising blood flow to the entire ipsilateral scrotum [12,28–30]. Although the timing of injury is often unclear, these torsions usually occur in utero [31–33], with the newborn presenting with a firm, discolored scrotum that is usually painless.

Although usually unilateral, bilateral perinatal torsion does occur [32,34,35]. The testis is usually necrotic at birth so that surgical salvage is rare [12]. In utero extravaginal torsion is not a surgical emergency, and some question if surgery is justified at all. In the uncommon case in which extravaginal torsion occurs after birth or produces only partial ischemia, the testis may be viable and hence salvageable with surgery [12,34]. Differential diagnostic considerations of a swollen scrotum in the

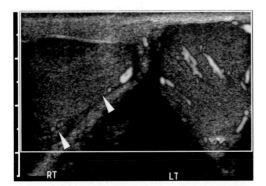

Fig. 4. Partial or incomplete testicular torsion. Transverse power Doppler sonogram shows minimal intratesticular blood flow (*arrowheads*) within the painful right testis, confirmed on other images. The amount of flow is clearly reduced, however, compared with the normal left testis. At operation, a viable testis with a 360° twist was salvaged.

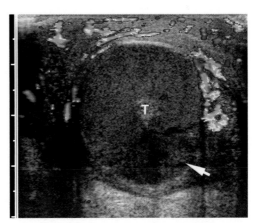

Fig. 6. Late testicular torsion. Transverse color Doppler sonogram of the left testis in a boy with 4 days of pain shows scrotal skin thickening and increased vascularity with an avascular testis (T). The testis has areas of heterogeneity (*arrow*) indicating infarction.

neonate include meconium peritonitis, intraperitoneal hemorrhage, tumor, hydrocele, and hernia.

If recently torsed, the testis appears enlarged and heterogeneous at sonography [36]. More commonly the chronically torsed testis is nearly normal in size and there is a peripheral echogenic rim corresponding to calcifications in the tunica albuginea, indicating a more remote event (Fig. 7). Color Doppler flow is absent in the testis and spermatic cord. In these small testes, power Doppler may be needed to detect blood flow even in normal testes [34]. If not recognized after birth, these testes gradually atrophy and may become calcified [36]. Small ovoid nubbins of tissue are sometimes found in the evaluation for unilateral cryptorchidism and presumably represent old perinatal torsions. The contralateral testis may demonstrate compensatory hypertrophy [35], a finding seen in other cases of congenital monorchidism [37].

Appendiceal torsion

Torsion of a testicular or epididymal appendage is the most common cause of acute scrotal pain in children before puberty, accounting for 26% to 67% of patients presenting to pediatric emergency departments [2,4,7,8,38–40]. This is probably an underestimate, because appendiceal torsion may account for most cases of prepubertal "epididymitis," because most children do not have any anatomic or infectious predisposition for true epididymitis and the imaging findings can be similar [3]. The testicular appendages are embryologic remnants [41], with the appendix testis attached to the tunica albuginea of the superior testis, and the appendix epididymis located on the epididymal head. Both appendices are pedunculated, predisposing them to torsion. The appendix testis is present in 92% of males, and the appendix epididymis is present in 25% [12]; thus, the appendix testis is the more common one to torse.

Although appendiceal torsion may mimic testicular torsion, the onset of pain tends to be more gradual than with testicular torsion, and systemic symptoms are usually absent [9]. Tenderness at examination may be focal or diffuse but is commonly localized to the superior scrotum. With gentle traction on the scrotal skin, a small bluish discoloration can be observed (blue dot sign), which represents the torsed appendage. Differentiation from testicular torsion is important, because appendiceal torsion is not a surgical emergency and responds well to conservative management [40]. Atrophy of the appendage and resolution of symptoms with supportive care is the usual outcome. Persistently symptomatic appendages may require surgical removal for pain relief.

On sonography, the torsed appendix appears as a small hyper- or hypoechoic mass adjacent to the superior aspect of the testis or epididymis [39,42]. Most are greater than 5 mm [40]. Coronal or transverse scanning above the testis may facilitate diagnosis [39]. With careful examination the sensitivity of sonographic detection of appendiceal torsion approaches 90% [42]. Although the torsed appendage has no flow, it incites an intense inflammatory response in the adjacent tissues. Color Doppler imaging demonstrates marked hyperemia focally around the area of torsion or diffusely throughout the entire testis and epididymis [27,39,43] (Fig. 8). The ultrasound appearance can be dramatic, with severe swelling and edema, scrotal skin thickening, and a reactive hydrocele [39,42,44]. Later the torsed appendage may appear as a small hyperechoic or calcified structure adjacent to the testis or may even detach to become an intrascrotal loose body or scrotolith (Fig. 9).

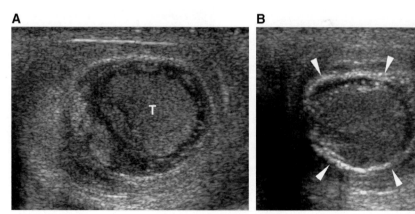

Fig. 7. Perinatal testicular torsion. (*A*) Sonogram in a newborn with a firm discolored scrotum shows the testis (T) surrounded by thickened scrotal soft tissues. No Doppler flow was demonstrable. (*B*) Sonogram performed 2 weeks later shows evolving calcifications within the tunica albuginea (*arrowheads*).

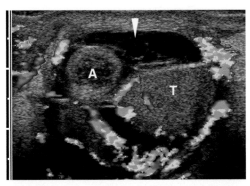

Fig. 8. Appendiceal torsion. Longitudinal color Doppler sonogram of the left scrotum shows an enlarged, heterogeneous, and avascular torsed appendage (A) with peritesticular hyperemia and increased flow to the testis (T). There is an associated hydrocele with septations (*arrowhead*).

Epididymitis and orchitis

Acute epididymitis

Although the exact incidence of acute epididymitis is unclear because of varying clinical and imaging diagnostic criteria among studies, epididymitis accounts for 28% to 47% of cases of acute scrotal pain among pediatric patients [4,7,8]. In fact, it is believed that many cases of prepubertal epididymitis (particularly those with negative urine cultures) are actually cases of appendiceal torsion [5,45]. Epididymitis is most common in the postpubertal adolescent.

As in adults, sexually transmitted disease and urinary tract infection are predisposing factors. The most common organisms are *Neisseria gonorrhoeae* and *Chlamydia trachomatis*, with *Escherichia coli* seen more commonly in younger boys [3]. In younger patients, noninfectious epididymitis can be caused by genitourinary abnormalities, such as an ectopic ureter draining into the vas deferens or seminal vesicles [12,46,47]. Physiologic or anatomic bladder outlet obstruction may lead to reflux of urine into the ejaculatory ducts, producing epididymitis. Epididymitis can occur after scrotal trauma [48] and it also may be idiopathic without a clear discernible etiology.

Clinically the onset of pain is more gradual than the other causes of the acute scrotum, and tenderness is often localized. Constitutional symptoms are uncommon. Presenting clinical findings are variable, ranging from mild scrotal tenderness without other complaints to severe scrotal edema, pain, and tenderness with fever and pyuria. In young patients, cultures are positive in 25% or fewer of cases [5,8,49].

Imaging reveals epididymal enlargement that may be diffuse or localized to one portion of the epididymis. The swollen epididymis is usually hypoechoic, but subsequent hemorrhage or edema can produce variable echogenicity. As with other inflammatory scrotal conditions, there is usually scrotal skin thickening and a reactive hydrocele.

Color Doppler shows increased blood flow in the inflamed epididymis compared with the asymptomatic side (Fig. 10). In most patients, the color Doppler findings confirm the gray-scale findings typical of scrotal inflammatory disease. In 20% of patients who have epididymitis, however, the gray-scale appearance of the epididymis is normal [50] and the inflammation is only revealed with color Doppler. With newer color Doppler technology, the normal epididymis shows minimal detectable flow [51], and the detection of any significant vascularity should be considered abnormal [3]. As with examination of the testes, comparing the amount of color

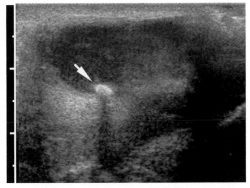

Fig. 9. Scrotolith. Transverse sonogram in a patient who had a prior history of a torsed appendage shows a calcification (*arrow*) that was freely mobile within the scrotum.

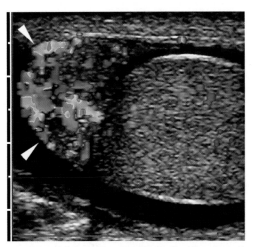

Fig. 10. Epididymitis. Longitudinal color Doppler sonogram in a teenager who had gonorrhea shows an enlarged and hyperemic epididymis (*arrowheads*), scrotal skin thickening, and a reactive hydrocele.

flow between the symptomatic and asymptomatic sides is helpful in recognizing pathology.

Orchitis

The most common cause of an inflammatory orchitis is secondary spread of inflammation from epididymitis, occurring in approximately 20% of postpubertal cases [25]. In acute epididymo-orchitis, the testis is usually enlarged and diffusely hypoechoic, becoming increasingly heterogeneous over time as the inflammatory process continues [52]. Focal lesions are less common, but when they occur, they appear as hypoechoic lesions adjacent to areas of epididymal inflammation. Inflammatory foci are often ill defined and can appear mass-like. The clinical scenario, however, usually differentiates infection from tumor. Color Doppler shows increased blood flow to the inflamed testis, with markedly increased diastolic flow [50,53]. Similar to epididymitis, gray-scale sonography is normal in 10% to 40% of patients who have orchitis, only being reliably detected with color flow imaging [53,54].

Acute epididymitis or epididymo-orchitis may produce testicular ischemia if spermatic vessels are compressed by a swollen epididymis or spermatic cord. Compromise of the draining pampiniform venous plexus and lymphatics is likely more important in producing testicular ischemia than is involvement of the testicular artery [55,56]. The testis appears enlarged and heterogeneous and has decreased or absent color flow. Pulsed Doppler waveforms demonstrate diastolic flow reversal of arterial waveforms resulting from increased intratesticular impedance caused by decreased venous outflow and vascular congestion. Resultant infarction may involve the entire testis or may produce focal lesions.

Primary orchitis is less common than secondary epididymo-orchitis and is usually viral in origin. Testicular inflammation from mumps orchitis occurs in approximately 30% of infected postpubertal boys [12]. Involvement is commonly bilateral, producing enlarged and heterogeneous testes at sonography that are hyperemic with color Doppler [57] (Fig. 11). Testicular atrophy may result, and later fertility is probably reduced.

Trauma

Scrotal trauma is common in childhood. As the physical examination may be limited by pain and swelling, ultrasound plays an important role in evaluating for hematoceles, testicular hematoma, or the more severe testicular fracture or rupture.

Traumatic hematoceles are common and appear acutely as echogenic fluid collections. As the

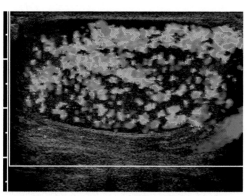

Fig. 11. Orchitis. Longitudinal sonogram in a boy who had a viral illness shows diffuse increased color Doppler flow.

hematoma organizes and clot retracts, the hematoma takes on the appearance of a complex septated cystic fluid collection (Fig. 12). Hematomas confined to the scrotal wall or peritesticular soft tissues also occur, and appear as variably echoic collections depending on their age.

Testicular hematoma results from blunt injury to the scrotum. As with hematomas elsewhere, the enlarged testis shows areas of increased or decreased parenchymal echogenicity depending on the age of the hematoma. Acutely, intratesticular hematomas are heterogeneous and may be hypo- or hyperechoic to surrounding testicular tissue (Fig. 13). Scrotal wall thickening and hydroceles or hematoceles are associated findings [3]. Color Doppler imaging is vital to prove viability of the traumatized

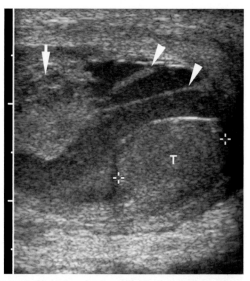

Fig. 12. Hematocele. Longitudinal sonogram 3 days after blunt scrotal trauma shows a normal testis (T) surrounded by echogenic fluid with early formation of organizing septations (*arrowheads*) and retracting clot (*arrow*).

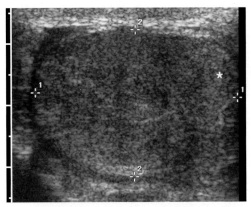

Fig. 13. Testicular hematoma. Transverse sonogram shows an enlarged testis with heterogeneous echotexture representing intratesticular hematoma. A small rim of normal parenchyma (*) is present.

testis and should show a normally perfused testis except for focal areas of absent vascularity in the area of the hematoma [27,58]. Follow-up imaging may reveal focal or diffuse testicular atrophy resulting from resorption of injured parenchyma or from ischemia from a surrounding hematocele or intratunica swelling [59].

Testicular fracture appears as a hypoechoic band interrupting the testicular parenchyma, but the testicular contour is well defined and the tunica albuginea is intact. A hematocele is common. Doppler evaluation is important. If perfusion to all portions of the testis can be identified, conservative management is possible; otherwise, emergent surgical exploration is required [60]. With testicular rupture, the hyperechoic tunica albuginea is interrupted, and there is extrusion of testicular tissue into the scrotum. This can be a difficult sonographic diagnosis, especially in the presence of a large hematocele. The testis appears heterogeneous because of hemorrhage and tissue injury and has ill-defined margins at the site of rupture [44,60]. Doppler rarely reveals flow, but surgery is indicated for attempted salvage and to remove any nonviable tissue that may lead to abscess formation or impede spermatogenesis in the remaining testis.

Varicocele

A varicocele is abnormal dilatation of the spermatic cord pampiniform venous plexus. There are two types: idiopathic (primary) and acquired (secondary). Most varicoceles in children are idiopathic, resulting from incompetent valves in the testicular veins. This allows retrograde blood flow into the pampiniform plexus and subsequent venous congestion and distension. The incidence of idiopathic varicoceles is 10% to 35% [61]; most are found in

adolescents and young adults and are more common on the left than the right side. The less common secondary varicoceles result from compression of the spermatic vein by a retroperitoneal mass or increased intra-abdominal pressure.

Patients usually present with more chronic complaints of dull scrotal pain or a feeling of heaviness, although symptoms may be more acute. Large varicoceles may be clinically visible as serpiginous venous structures along the scrotal wall and inguinal canal. Small varicoceles may be detectable by palpation, which is facilitated by having the patient stand upright or perform a Valsalva maneuver. There may be ipsilateral hypotrophy of the testis and reduced sperm quality, the degree of which correlates with the severity of the varicocele [62–64]. Treatment depends on the degree of symptoms and whether there are any testicular changes. Small varicoceles are usually treated. Large varicoceles may require repair to relieve symptoms and to allow normal testicular growth. Varicocele repair can be performed surgically or by transcatheter interventional embolization or sclerotherapy.

Sonographically, varicoceles appear as tortuous, anechoic structures within the superior scrotum, which may extend along the length of the testis. Venous diameters can range between 2 and 7 mm, in contrast to normal vein diameters of 0.5 to 2 mm. Varicoceles increase in size and show augmented color Doppler flow with the patient upright or performing the Valsalva maneuver [58,65] (Fig. 14).

Inguinal hernia

Inguinal hernias are common scrotal masses in young patients and are almost always indirect hernias resulting from a patent processus vaginalis. These hernias are more common on the right, because the right processus vaginalis closes after the left during development. Most hernias are clinically obvious, but sonography can be useful in patients who present with scrotal enlargement of unknown cause. Hernias may contain small bowel, colon, or omentum.

Patients present with chronic or acute complaints of swelling and groin pain. Abdominal pain and vomiting may occur, which may indicate incarceration or strangulation of hernia contents. Physical examination discloses scrotal swelling that extends along the inguinal canal. Often hernias are reducible with gentle upward pressure, providing relief of symptoms and confirming the diagnosis. If irreducible, or if the patient has too much discomfort to tolerate reduction attempts, ultrasound can be used to confirm the diagnosis before more aggressive treatment is instituted.

A   **B**

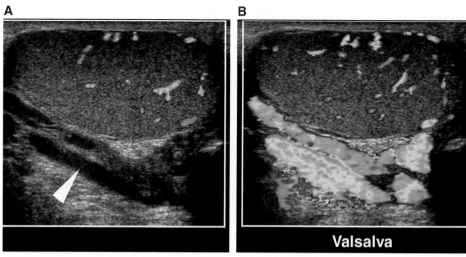

Fig. 14. Varicocele. Longitudinal color Doppler sonogram of the left scrotum at rest (*A*) shows dilated veins with internal echoes representing slow venous flow (*arrowhead*) but no color Doppler signal. With Valsalva (*B*), the veins distend and there is marked color Doppler flow.

Bowel is easily characterized by ultrasound, and a hernia is definitively diagnosed by demonstrating bowel within the inguinal canal and scrotum (Fig. 15), with a normal testis and epididymis. Omental hernias may be more difficult to recognize, appearing as a complex echogenic mass [44]. This appearance is nonspecific and can overlap with other masses or complex collections, but may be suspected from the increased echogenicity caused by fat and the presence of parallel omental vessels. If bowel is identified, observing peristalsis indicates viability, whereas lack of peristalsis or the presence of submucosal hemorrhage and edema indicates ischemic injury.

It is not enough to just scan the patient lying quietly. Identifying a hernia often requires raising the

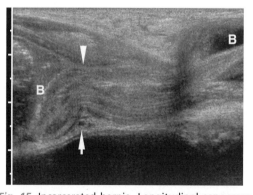

Fig. 15. Incarcerated hernia. Longitudinal sonogram through the right inguinal canal shows bowel (B) extending from the abdominal cavity through an enlarged internal inguinal ring (*arrowhead*) into the scrotum. Arrow marks the inferior epigastric artery. The hernia was not reducible, but the hernia contents were viable at surgery.

intra-abdominal pressure by having the patient Valsalva or stand upright to bring the hernia into view. The inferior epigastric artery is a useful landmark for identifying the internal inguinal ring [66,67] (Fig. 15). A canal width of greater than 4 mm at the internal ring has a sensitivity of 95% in diagnosing a hernia [67].

Hydrocele

Hydroceles are common causes of scrotal swelling. Although usually painless, they may occasionally present with pain or diffuse discomfort. In infants and young children, hydroceles are almost always caused by peritoneal fluid extending through a patent processus vaginalis [68]. In older patients, hydroceles may result from inflammatory processes, testicular or appendiceal torsion, trauma, or tumors. In these cases, the degree of pain associated with a hydrocele often depends on the coexisting abnormality.

If large, hydroceles can make palpation of the scrotal contents difficult or impossible. Transillumination of the scrotum may help to confirm the presence of a hydrocele but does little to evaluate for any associated pathology. Sonography greatly assists in this evaluation.

At sonography, hydroceles are typically thin-walled fluid collections that typically surround the anterior surface of the testis (Fig. 16). If hydrocele fluid completely surrounds the testis, a bell-clapper deformity exists and the child is at risk for testicular torsion. If the processes vaginalis closes superiorly and inferiorly, a hydrocele may present as an encysted collection within the spermatic cord. Least common is the abdominoscrotal hydrocele, which

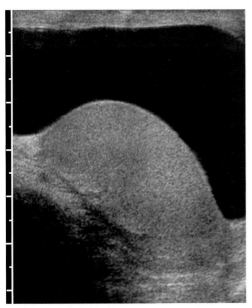

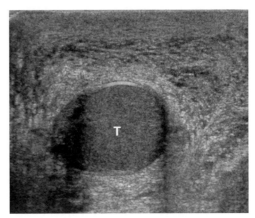

Fig. 17. Idiopathic scrotal edema. Transverse sonogram shows marked thickening of the scrotal wall. The testis (T) is entirely normal.

Fig. 16. Hydrocele. Longitudinal sonogram shows anechoic fluid surrounding the anterior aspect of the testis, which is fixed posteriorly to the scrotal wall.

presents as a scrotal and pelvic mass [69]. Hydrocele fluid is most often anechoic [44,68] but can contain internal echoes from hemorrhage, infection, or cholesterol crystals [44,68]. More chronic hydroceles may have a thicker wall, and scrotoliths may form within the fluid.

Idiopathic scrotal edema

Idiopathic scrotal edema produces scrotal enlargement usually in patients younger than 10 years of age, with most being between the ages of 4 and 7 years. Patients present with mild scrotal tenderness, swelling, and erythema [12]. The scrotal contents are normal to palpation. Clinically the condition resembles a cellulitis or reaction to an insect bite, but there is no break in the skin or other evidence of infection.

At sonography, the scrotal soft tissues are thickened and edematous (Fig. 17). The scrotal wall is hypoechoic with echogenic septae that show flow with color Doppler. There is often diffuse color Doppler hyperemia of the scrotum. The testis and epididymis are completely normal [26,58]. Acute scrotal edema resolves spontaneously within several days with symptomatic treatment and without sequelae [12].

Henoch-Schönlein purpura

Any vasculitis can potentially involve the scrotum, but in children it is usually caused by Henoch-Schönlein purpura (HSP). HSP is a small vessel vasculitis involving multiple organ systems, especially the skin, gastrointestinal tract, kidneys, and joints. The scrotum is involved in 15% to 38% of cases, occasionally before the involvement of other systems is clinically apparent [70,71]. The clinical picture is usually sufficient for diagnosis, but scrotal pain may prompt imaging to insure that no other pathology is present.

Sonographically the testes are typically normal. The epididymides, however, are usually enlarged and heterogeneous, and there is often a reactive hydrocele and scrotal skin thickening (Fig. 18). Color Doppler imaging shows epididymal hyperemia and inflammation but normal intratesticular flow [70,71].

Summary

Various conditions may present as an acute scrotum in children. The combination of history, physical examination, and imaging results can often pinpoint a correct diagnosis, which expedites appropriate patient care. Ultrasound is the most useful diagnostic

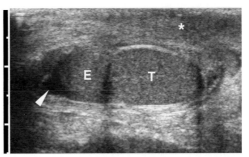

Fig. 18. Henoch-Schönlein purpura. Longitudinal sonogram shows an enlarged epididymis (E) and a normal testis (T). There is thickening of the scrotal skin (*) and a small reactive hydrocele (*arrowhead*).

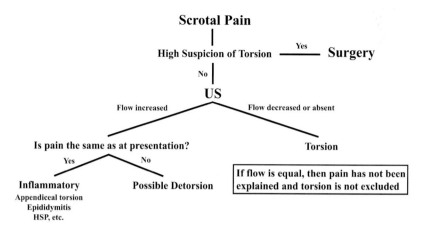

Fig. 19. Suggested algorithm for the approach to pediatric scrotal pain. The importance of the clinical examination is paramount.

modality, allowing detailed gray-scale anatomic assessment and providing information about blood flow and perfusion with color Doppler. With the current sensitivity of color Doppler, the diagnosis of testicular torsion is no longer a binary decision, and the status of the patient's pain at the time of imaging must also be taken into consideration. Fig. 19 shows a suggested algorithm. Although no diagnostic examination is completely free from error, careful technique and an understanding of those conditions producing acute scrotal pain in children should improve diagnostic accuracy.

References

[1] Karmazyn B, Steinberg R, Kornreich L, et al. Clinical and sonographic criteria of acute scrotum in children: a retrospective study of 172 boys. Pediatr Radiol 2005;35:302–10.

[2] Lam W, Yap T, Jacobsen A, et al. Colour Doppler ultrasonography replacing surgical exploration for acute scrotum: myth or reality? Pediatr Radiol 2005;35:597–600.

[3] Coley BD, Siegel MJ. Male genital tract. In: Siegel MJ, editor. Pediatric sonography. 3rd edition. Philadelphia: Lippincott, Williams & Wilkins; 2002. p. 579–624.

[4] Campobasso P, Donadio P, Spata E, et al. Acute scrotum in pediatric age: analysis of 265 consecutive cases. Pediatr Med Chir 1996;18:15–20.

[5] Kadish HA, Bolte RG. A retrospective review of pediatric patients with epididymitis, testicular torsion, and torsion of testicular appendages. Pediatrics 1998;102:73–6.

[6] Kass EJ, Stone KT, Cacciarelli AA, et al. Do all children with an acute scrotum require exploration? J Urol 1993;150:667–9.

[7] Lewis AG, Bukowski TP, Jarvis PD, et al. Evaluation of acute scrotum in the emergency department. J Pediatr Surg 1995;30:277–82.

[8] Sidler D, Brown RA, Millar AJ, et al. A 25-year review of the acute scrotum in children. S Afr Med J 1997;87:1696–8.

[9] Jefferson RH, Perez LM, Joseph DB. Critical analysis of the clinical presentation of acute scrotum: a 9-year experience at a single institution. J Urol 1997;158:1198–200.

[10] Ciftci A, Senocak M, Tanyeo F, et al. Clinical predictors for differential diagnosis of acute scrotum. Eur J Pediatr Surg 2004;14:333–8.

[11] Garel L, Dubois J, Azzie G, et al. Preoperative manual detorsion of the spermatic cord with Doppler ultrasound monitoring in patients with intravaginal acute testicular torsion. Pediatr Radiol 2000;30:41–4.

[12] Kogan S, Hadziselimovic F, Howards SS, et al. Pediatric andrology. In: Gillenwater JY, Grayhack JT, Howards SS, et al, editors. Adult and pediatric urology. 3rd edition. St. Louis: Mosby; 1996. p. 2623–74.

[13] Mendel JB, Taylor GA, Treves S, et al. Testicular torsion in children: scintigraphic assessment. Pediatr Radiol 1985;15:110–5.

[14] Prando D. Torsion of the spermatic cord: sonographic diagnosis. Ultrasound Q 2002;18:41–57.

[15] Kalfa N, Veyrac C, Baud C, et al. Ultrasonography of the spermatic cord in children with testicular torsion: impact on the surgical strategy. J Urol 2004;172:1692–5.

[16] Baud C, Veyrac C, Couture A, et al. Spiral twist of the spermatic cord: a reliable sign of testicular torsion. Pediatr Radiol 1998;28:950–4.

[17] Orazi C, Schingo P, Ferro F, et al. Does B-mode ultrasound still have a role in the diagnosis of spermatic cord torsion? Findings in a pediatric series. Radiol Med (Torino) 1997;94:646–51.

[18] Arce JD, Cortes M, Vargas JC. Sonographic diagnosis of acute spermatic cord torsion: rotation of the cord, a key to the diagnosis. Pediatr Radiol 2002;32:485–91.

[19] Middleton WD, Middleton MA, Dierks M, et al. Sonographic prediction of viability in testicular

torsion: preliminary observations. J Ultrasound Med 1997;16:23–7.

[20] Burks DD, Markey BJ, Burkhard TK, et al. Suspected testicular torsion and ischemia: evaluation with color Doppler sonography. Radiology 1990;175:815–21.

[21] Siegel MJ. The acute scrotum. Radiol Clin North Am 1997;35:959–76.

[22] Steinhardt GF, Boyarsky S, Mackey R. Testicular torsion: pitfalls of color Doppler sonography. J Urol 1993;150:461–2.

[23] Wilbert DM, Schaerfe CW, Stern WD, et al. Evaluation of the acute scrotum by color-coded Doppler ultrasonography. J Urol 1993;149:1475–7.

[24] Dogra V, Sessions A, Mevorach R, et al. Reversal of diastolic plateau in partial testicular torsion. J Clin Ultrasound 2001;29:105–8.

[25] Gronski M, Hollman AS. The acute paediatric scrotum: the role of colour Doppler ultrasound. Eur J Radiol 1998;26:183–93.

[26] Grainger AJ, Hide IG, Elliott ST. The ultrasound appearances of scrotal oedema. Eur J Ultrasound 1998;8:33–7.

[27] Lerner RM, Mevorach RA, Hulbert WC, et al. Color Doppler US in the evaluation of acute scrotal disease. Radiology 1990;176:355–8.

[28] Patriquin HB, Yazbeck S, Trinh B, et al. Testicular torsion in infants and children: diagnosis with Doppler sonography. Radiology 1993;188:781–5.

[29] Leape LL. Torsion of the testis. In: Welch KJ, Randolph JG, Ravitch MM, et al, editors. Pediatric surgery. Chicago: Year Book; 1986. p. 1330–4.

[30] Brown SM, Casillas VJ, Montalvo BM, et al. Intrauterine spermatic cord torsion in the newborn: sonographic and pathologic correlation. Radiology 1990;177:755–7.

[31] Devesa R, Munoz A, Torrents M, et al. Prenatal diagnosis of testicular torsion. [see comments]. Ultrasound Obstet Gynecol 1998;11:286–8.

[32] Groisman GM, Nassrallah M, Bar-Maor JA. Bilateral intra-uterine testicular torsion in a newborn. Br J Urol 1996;78:800–1.

[33] Youssef BA, Sammak BM, Al Shahed M. Case report. Pre-natally diagnosed testicular torsion ultrasonographic features. Clin Radiol 2000;55:150–1.

[34] Zinn HL, Cohen HL, Horowitz M. Testicular torsion in neonates: importance of power Doppler imaging. J Ultrasound Med 1998;17:385–8.

[35] Cartwright PC, Snow BW, Reid BS, et al. Color Doppler ultrasound in newborn testis torsion. Urology 1995;45:667–70.

[36] Traubici J, Daneman A, Navarro O, et al. Testicular torsion in neonates and infants: sonographic features in 30 patients. Am J Roentgenol 2003;180:1143–5.

[37] Koff SA. Does compensatory testicular enlargement predict monorchism? J Urol 1991;146:632–3.

[38] Atkinson GO Jr, Patrick LE, Ball TI Jr, et al. The normal and abnormal scrotum in children: evaluation with color Doppler sonography. Am J Roentgenol 1992;158:613–7.

[39] Strauss S, Faingold R, Manor H. Torsion of the testicular appendages: sonographic appearance. J Ultrasound Med 1997;16:189–92.

[40] Baldisserotto M, de Souza L, Pertence A, et al. Color Doppler sonography of normal and torsed testicular appendages in children. Am J Roentgenol 2005;184:1287–92.

[41] Black JA, Patel A. Sonography of the normal extratesticular space. Am J Roentgenol 1996;167:503–6.

[42] Hesser U, Rosenborg M, Gierup J, et al. Grayscale sonography in torsion of the testicular appendages. Pediatr Radiol 1993;23:529–32.

[43] Monga M, Scarpero HM, Ortenberg J. Metachronous bilateral torsion of the testicular appendices. Int J Urol 1999;6:589–91.

[44] Hill MC, Sanders RC. Sonography of benign disease of the scrotum. In: Sanders RC, Hill MC, editors. Ultrasound annual. New York: Raven Press; 1986. p. 197–237.

[45] Kass EJ, Lundak B. The acute scrotum. Pediatr Clin North Am 1997;44:1251–66.

[46] Bukowski TP, Lewis AG, Reeves D, et al. Epididymitis in older boys: dysfunctional voiding as an etiology. J Urol 1995;154:762–5.

[47] Siegel A, Snyder H, Duckett JW. Epididymitis in infants and boys: underlying urogenital anomalies and efficacy of imaging modalities. J Urol 1987;138:1100–3.

[48] Gordon LM, Stein SM, Ralls PW. Traumatic epididymitis: evaluation with color Doppler sonography. Am J Roentgenol 1996;166:1323–5.

[49] Lau P, Anderson PA, Giacomantonio JM, et al. Acute epididymitis in boys: are antibiotics indicated? Br J Urol 1997;79:797–800.

[50] Horstman WG, Middleton WD, Melson GL, et al. Scrotal inflammatory disease: color Doppler US findings. Radiology 1991;179:55–9.

[51] Luker GD, Siegel MJ. Scrotal US in pediatric patients: comparison of power and standard color Doppler US. Radiology 1996;198:381–5.

[52] Cook JL, Dewbury K. The changes seen on high-resolution ultrasound in orchitis. Clin Radiol 2000;55:13–8.

[53] Jee WH, Choe BY, Byun JY, et al. Resistive index of the intrascrotal artery in scrotal inflammatory disease. Acta Radiol 1997;38:1026–30.

[54] Middleton WD, Siegel BA, Melson GL, et al. Acute scrotal disorders: prospective comparison of color Doppler US and testicular scintigraphy. Radiology 1990;177:177–81.

[55] Sue SR, Pelucio M, Gibbs M. Testicular infarction in a patient with epididymitis. Acad Emerg Med 1998;5:1128–30.

[56] Chin SC, Wu CJ, Chen A, et al. Segmental hemorrhagic infarction of testis associated with epididymitis. J Clin Ultrasound 1998;26:326–8.

[57] Tarantino L, Giorgio A, de Stefano G, et al. Echo color Doppler findings in postpubertal mumps epididymo-orchitis. J Ultrasound Med 2001;20:1189–95.

[58] Luker GD, Siegel MJ. Color Doppler sonography of the scrotum in children. Am J Roentgenol 1994;163:649–55.

[59] Cross JJ, Berman LH, Elliott PG, et al. Scrotal trauma: a cause of testicular atrophy. Clin Radiol 1999;54:317–20.

[60] Hricak H, Hamm B, Kim B. Imaging of the scrotum: textbook and atlas. New York: Raven Press; 1995.

[61] Nagar H, Mabjeesh NJ. Decision-making in pediatric varicocele surgery: use of color Doppler ultrasound. Pediatr Surg Int 2000;16:75–6.

[62] Lund L, Tang YC, Roebuck D, et al. Testicular catch-up growth after varicocele correction in adolescents. Pediatr Surg Int 1999;15:234–7.

[63] Sayfan J, Siplovich L, Koltun L, et al. Varicocele treatment in pubertal boys prevents testicular growth arrest. J Urol 1997;157:1456–7.

[64] Zini A, Buckspan M, Beradinucci D, et al. Loss of left testicular volume in men with clinical left varicocele: correlation with grade of varicocele. Arch Androl 1998;41:37–41.

[65] Cornud F, Belin X, Amar E, et al. Varicocele: strategies in diagnosis and treatment. Eur Radiol 1999;9:536–45.

[66] Korenkov M, Paul A, Troidl H. Color duplex sonography: diagnostic tool in the differentiation of inguinal hernias. J Ultrasound Med 1999;18:565–8.

[67] Chen KC, Chu CC, Chou TY, et al. Ultrasonography for inguinal hernias in boys. J Pediatr Surg 1998;33:1784–7.

[68] Chung SE, Frush DP, Fordham LA. Sonographic appearances of extratesticular fluid and fluid-containing scrotal masses in infants and children: clues to diagnosis. Am J Roentgenol 1999;173:741–5.

[69] Fenton L, McCabe K. Giant unilateral abdominoscrotal hydrocele. Pediatr Radiol 2002; 32:882–4.

[70] Sudakoff GS, Burke M, Rifkin MD. Ultrasonographic and color Doppler imaging of hemorrhagic epididymitis in Henoch-Schönlein purpura. J Ultrasound Med 1992;11:619–21.

[71] Ben-Sira L, Laor T. Severe scrotal pain in boys with Henoch-Schönlein purpura: incidence and sonography. Pediatr Radiol 2000;30:125–8.

ULTRASOUND CLINICS

Ultrasound Clin 1 (2006) 497–507

The Painful Extremity

Sabah Servaes, MD*, Richard Bellah, MD

- Technique
- Trauma
- Infection/inflammation
- Low-flow vascular malformations
- Summary
- Acknowledgments
- References

Sonography has distinct advantages over every other modality in regard to musculoskeletal imaging of pediatric patients. A review of its usefulness in assessment of the painful extremity includes traumatic, infectious, inflammatory, and developmental etiologies.

The most common use of musculoskeletal ultrasound in pediatric imaging is the evaluation of developmental dysplasia of the hip, but the potential role of ultrasound in evaluation of the pediatric musculoskeletal system is much more far-reaching. Image quality, radiation exposure, and cost factor into the decision of which imaging study serves patients best. Although MR imaging uses no ionizing radiation and provides excellent visualization of soft tissues and marrow edema, its cost, availability, and need for sedation are drawbacks. Sonography provides excellent imaging in patients who are skeletally immature, is readily available, can be obtained portably and without sedation, and can be performed dynamically to address clinical questions most effectively. This article reviews the use of sonography in the evaluation of the painful extremity of pediatric patients.

Technique

A high-frequency linear array transducer is used most frequently when performing pediatric musculoskeletal sonographic examinations. Imaging performed in two orthogonal planes can be done to delineate the anatomy and pathologic processes. The dynamic examination, which may incorporate oblique planes, allows the examiner to assess movement of joints. Comparison with the contralateral, asymptomatic side provides a useful standard to identify normal anatomy. The addition of duplex Doppler may provide additional information regarding inflammation.

Trauma

Radiography is the usual first choice for imaging musculoskeletal injury. Sonography can be an excellent complement to evaluate the soft tissues or cartilage, particularly in patients who are skeletally immature.

Sonography is a sensitive method to evaluate myotendinous insult from traction injury or muscular contusion and tear from direct impact [1,2]. Sonography of a myotendinous tear demonstrates discontinuity of the tissues often with fluid accumulation [2–4]. Intramuscular tear and contusion are recognized by loss of the normal muscular architecture and the presence of blood. Heterogeneity of blood products may be visualized in a variety of phases of organization, depending on the time of imaging relative to injury (Fig. 1). Follow-up sonographic examination is advised to ensure resolution and that no underlying pathologic process exists that might have led to the hemorrhage.

The Children's Hospital of Philadelphia, 34th and Civic Center Boulevard, Philadelphia, PA 19104, USA
* Corresponding author.
E-mail address: servaes@email.chop.edu (S. Servaes).

1556-858X/06/$ – see front matter © 2006 Elsevier Inc. All rights reserved.
ultrasound.theclinics.com

doi:10.1016/j.cult.2006.05.009

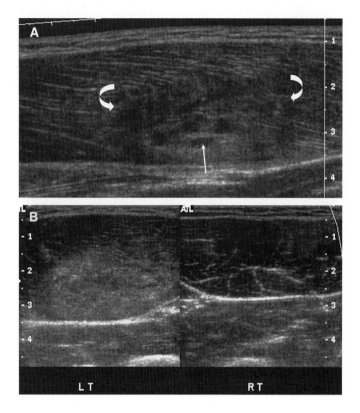

Fig. 1. Intramuscular contusion and tear. (*A*) Sagittal sonogram of the symptomatic, left rectus femorus demonstrates increased echogenicity and disruption of the muscle fibers representing an intramuscular tear and contusion (*curved arrows*) and anechoic fluid within the substance of the muscle. The straight arrow points to fluid within the substance of the rectus femorus muscle. (*B*) Transverse sonogram through the rectus femorus bilaterally demonstrating the increased echogenicity and increased width of the left (LT) muscle compared with the normal right (RT).

Hemophiliacs are at increased risk of painful bleeding into joints or within muscles, and sonography provides an effective method to identify synovial and intramuscular involvement (Fig. 2). The hinge joints (knee and elbow) are the most common sites of intra-articular hemorrhage, but the wrist, shoulder, hand, foot, and hip also can be affected. Intramuscular hemorrhage occurs most commonly in the iliopsoas and, less commonly, in the rectus abdominus muscle and retroperitoneum [5]. Degenerative joint disease can occur after multiple episodes of intra-articular hemorrhage but is evaluated best with radiographs.

In nonaccidental trauma, ultrasound can provide information regarding the integrity of surrounding soft tissue structures and can clarify equivocal radiologic findings, such as an indefinite metaphyseal fracture [6–8]. If a radiologic finding suggests an

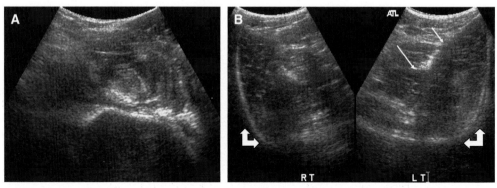

Fig. 2. (*A*) Iliacus hemorrhage in a patient who had hemophilia; echogenic curvilinear line is the iliac bone. (*B*) Comparison view of the asymptomatic right side (RT) is on the left side of the image and the symptomatic left side (LT) is to the right. Straight arrows point to the iliacus hemorrhage on the patient's left. Double-headed arrows point to iliac bones.

osseous abnormality, ultrasound may be useful in further assessment of the clinical question by identifying associated soft tissue injury (Fig. 3).

Epiphyseal injury (which may result from birth trauma) can be radiographically occult but is identified readily with ultrasound. The ossification centers of the proximal humerus and the capitellum are not apparent radiographically at birth or for several months of life [9,10]. Epiphyseal separation is difficult to diagnose on conventional radiography, because the location of the epiphysis cannot be inferred easily from the radiographs. Ultrasound of an epiphyseal separation shows discontinuity between the epiphysis and metaphysis, whereas the relationship of the unossified articular surfaces remains well preserved. Ultrasound also can be used to distinguish between a fracture at the proximal or distal physis of the humerus versus a dislocation.

In adolescents, traction injury at the ends of the patellar tendon can result in Sinding-Larsen-Johansson disease or Osgood-Schlatter disease.

Sinding-Larsen-Johansson disease is a subset of jumper's knee (seen in individuals who are skeletally mature), which typically results from repetitive trauma in activities, including jumping, kicking, and running. In Sinding-Larsen-Johansson disease, the affected site is the inferior pole of the patella at the origin of the patellar tendon. Sonographically, the patellar tendon appears enlarged and hyperechoic and may contain ossific fragments. The adjacent soft tissues are edematous. Osgood-Schlatter disease involves the tendon insertion at the tibial tuberosity and often is diagnosed clinically. The patellar tendon is thickened and there is adjacent edema of the cartilage and soft tissues. Grading of these injuries is based largely on clinical criteria, with the most severe level corresponding to complete disruption of fibers. The incidence of bilateral disease with Osgood-Schlatter disease is 25% [11].

Baker's cysts in children may develop secondary to trauma or synovitis. Baker's cysts are fluid collections between the medial head of the gastrocnemius

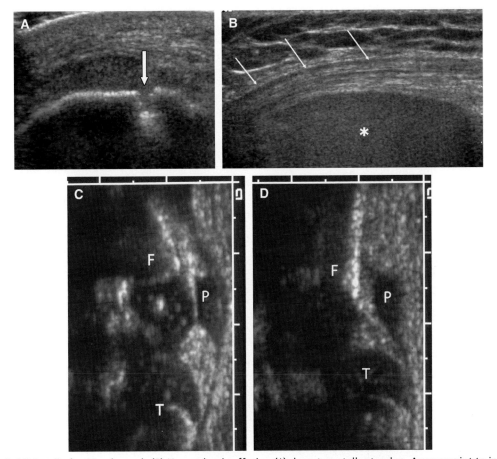

Fig. 3. (*A*) Patella fracture (*arrow*). (*B*) Hemorrhagic effusion (***) deep to patellar tendon. Arrows point to intact patellar tendon. (*C*) Normal knee. (*D*) Dislocated knee the tibia displaced anterior relative to the femur (F). P, patella; T, tibia.

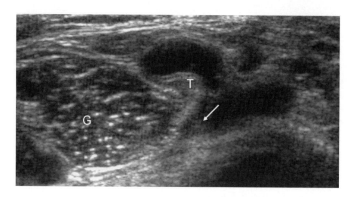

Fig. 4. Baker's cyst. Lobulated anechoic mass in the popliteal fossa is a Baker's cyst. The neck of the cyst (*arrow*) insinuates between the tendon of the gastrocnemius muscle (G) overlies the gastrocnemius muscle and T marks the gastrocnemius tendon and semimembranosis.

and semimembranosus tendons. These cysts usually are found incidentally but can be associated with pain if they rupture, leak, or compress other structures [12]. Ultrasound is excellent at detecting the cysts, with accuracies reported at 100% [13]. In children, ultrasound is a simple method to assure that a mass in the popliteal fossa is cystic in nature. Sonographically, Baker's cysts are hypoechoic, occasionally septated, well-defined masses found in the medial aspect of the popliteal fossa (Fig. 4). Baker's cysts arise less frequently in children than in adults and typically resolve spontaneously [14]. In cases associated with synovitis, it is prudent to scan the suprapatellar region to evaluate for other evidence of joint disease.

Infection and inflammation

Sonography demonstrates abnormalities in a variety of musculoskeletal infections, including cellulitis, necrotizing fasciitis, bursitis, tenosynovitis, myositis, arthritis, and osteomyelitis [15–19]. The findings of cellulitis (subcutaneous inflammation) include increased echogenicity, thickening of tissues (including skin), loss of tissue planes, and insinuating fluid (Fig. 5). Color Doppler demonstrates increased flow to the area distinguishing cellulitis from edema [19]. An infection within the soft tissues can become walled off to form an abscess, which can be identified easily with ultrasound and drained with ultrasound guidance. An abscess usually is round or ovoid, can demonstrate varying degrees of echogenicity depending on contents, and has increased through transmission. There should be no demonstrable Doppler flow within an abscess, and there may be hyperemia of the wall [19]. Sonography also can help distinguish between an abscess and enlarged lymph nodes (Fig. 6). Patients who have sickle cell disease are shown to have frequent soft tissue infections, which clinically may simulate bone marrow infarction [17]. Sonographic assessment and distinction in these patients, therefore, can have a significant impact on patient care. The ultrasound findings of necrotizing fasciitis are similar to cellulitis, but the sensitivity and specificity are not reported; radiography and CT, therefore, remain the modalities of choice to recognize air in the subcutaneous tissues.

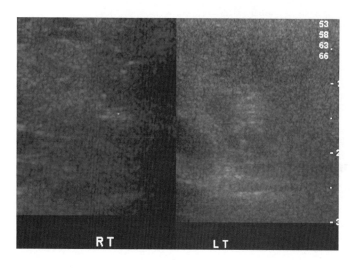

Fig. 5. Cellulitis. Note the increased echogenicity on the symptomatic left (LT) side.

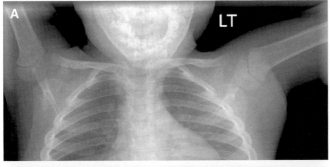

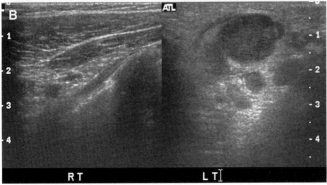

Fig. 6. Lymphadenopathy. (*A*) Frontal chest radiograph demonstrating mass at left axilla. (*B*) Split-screen ultrasound image showing left (LT) axillary lymphadenopathy with the normal right axilla (RT) for comparison.

Myositis, bursitis, and tenosynovitis sonographically appear as increased echogenicity within and surrounding the corresponding inflamed tissue (Fig. 7) [19]. Myositis can be similar in appearance to intramuscular contusion, rendering clinical history, response to therapy, and follow-up imaging important. The sonographic findings in bursitis include thickening of the wall of the bursa and surrounding fluid [11]. Tenosynovitis is evidenced at ultrasound by an enlarged tendon with surrounding fluid within the tendon sheath (Fig. 8). Color flow Doppler occasionally may demonstrate

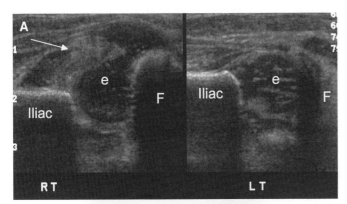

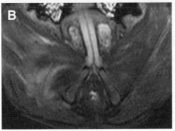

Fig. 7. Myositis. (*A*) Coronal ultrasound of the hips comparing both sides. The infant maintained the right hip in flexion and had a history of staphylococcal infection. The ultrasound was performed to evaluate for dislocation. The femoral heads (e) are well seated in the acetabula (Iliac), but there is thickening and increased echogenicity of the adjacent soft tissues (*arrow*) on the right (RT) compared with the left (LT). (*B*) Axial T2-weighted MR image with fat saturation demonstrates increased abnormal signal about the right hip. F, femoral metaphysis.

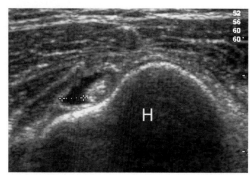

Fig. 8. Biceps tendon inflammation with fluid surrounding the tendon (marked by calipers) and humerus (H).

hyperemia [20]. Comparison with the contralateral side is especially helpful.

Arthritis may be infectious or inflammatory in etiology. Juvenile rheumatoid arthritis is the most common cause of noninfectious joint inflammation. The large joints typically are involved, with the knee affected most frequently. Sonographic evaluation focuses on evaluation of the synovial thickening, effusion, and soft tissue swelling [21–24]. Proliferative synovium is thick, irregular, and hyperechoic and demonstrates increased Doppler flow. The synovium of the knee is seen best in the suprapatellar bursa, but it always is important to search posteriorly for associated Baker's cysts (Fig. 9). Evaluation of therapeutic response on synovial hyperemia is shown with power Doppler sonography [25]. These findings can be seen before the articular changes, which appear radiographically. The majority of pediatric patients who have rheumatoid arthritis are seronegative. Exclusion of a septic joint, therefore, often is necessary in children who present with a swollen and painful joint with an effusion. In the latter instance, ultrasound is suited to guide aspiration.

Children who present with a painful hip are a clinical and diagnostic challenge. The differential diagnosis includes septic hip, toxic synovitis, Legg-

Calvé-Perthes disease, and slipped capital femoral epiphysis. Radiographs with the hips in neutral and frog-leg lateral positions may be all that is required to diagnose Legg-Calvé-Perthes disease and slipped capital femoral epiphysis. Ultrasound also can demonstrate, however, the epiphyseal changes in patients who have Legg-Calvé-Perthes disease (Fig. 10), and contrast-enhanced power Doppler sonography is shown effective for depiction of the revascularization process, particularly within the physis [26].

Hip joint effusions are difficult to evaluate radiographically, particularly when small, but sonography is an excellent modality in the evaluation of hip joint effusion [27–29]. An anterior parasagittal plane parallel to the femoral neck with the hips extended is the best approach to detect an effusion, because the anterior capsular space is where an effusion is most likely to accumulate [28]. The effusion is seen as a hypoechoic fluid layer between the anterior and posterior layers of the anterior joint capsule (Fig. 11A). Asymptomatic children may have some fluid within the joint, but fluid measuring greater than 2 mm is considered abnormal. Comparison with the contralateral side provides an internal control (see Fig. 11B). Abduction with the hip in extension maximizes visualization and is recommended in equivocal cases, but this position is more painful for patients because of the resultant increased intracapsular pressure [27].

Laboratory values and clinical signs may help distinguish between hip effusion resulting from toxic synovitis and a septic hip. Approximately half of patients who have toxic synovitis have a history of recent illness, ranging from upper respiratory infection to otitis media. Typically, children who have a septic hip have an elevated erythrocyte sedimentation rate (ESR), white blood count (WBC), C-reactive protein, and temperature in contradistinction to children who have toxic synovitis, but these findings may not be true early in the presentation of a septic hip and some elevation of these values may be seen with toxic synovitis. Kocher

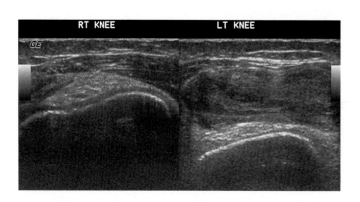

Fig. 9. Juvenile rheumatoid arthritis. Left knee suprapatellar complex effusion and contralateral normal right knee.

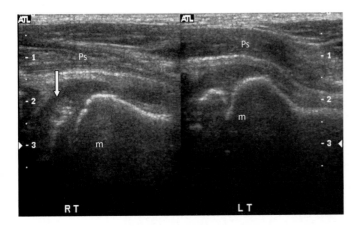

Fig. 10. Legg-Calvé-Perthes disease. Arrow points to flattened epiphysis of the right femur. m, femoral metaphysis; Ps, psoas muscle.

and colleagues identified a combination of four clinical predictors to help differentiate septic arthritis from transient synovitis: history of fever, history of non–weight bearing, ESR greater than 40 mm per hour, and serum WBC count greater than 12,000 cells per microliter [30]. With two of these predictors, the probability of septic arthritis is 40%, and sonography is helpful in deciding which patients require aspiration. Children who have three or more predictors have a probability of septic hip greater than 93% and usually require operative treatment instead of aspiration.

Because of the permanent sequelae, which may result from the untreated septic hip and the overlap of clinical presentation with toxic synovitis, some use Doppler sonography to help with the distinction between these two entities. Power Doppler or color Doppler may demonstrate increased flow in the septic hip, but the absence of increased flow does not exclude the diagnosis [31]. Similarly, the resistive index of the posterior capsule vessels may increase with large effusions [32]. Because a septic effusion may be present without abnormal

Doppler findings, aspiration is recommended in the appropriate clinical setting to exclude infection. Aspiration also is therapeutic by relieving increased intracapsular pressure, which constitutes an indication for tapping the joint in some cases of toxic synovitis [33] and provides symptomatic relief. Ultrasound is useful in guidance for hip aspiration procedures.

Osteomyelitis is common especially in the pediatric population. *Staphylococcus aureus* typically is the causative organism in the pediatric population (group B beta hemolytic streptococcus is second in neonates). Tubular bones are involved most commonly. MR imaging remains the most sensitive examination in the acute setting because of its ability to demonstrate bone marrow edema. Sonographic findings may become apparent within 1 to 2 days after symptoms and several days before radiographic changes [16]. This time frame is similar to that during which nuclear imaging demonstrates osteomyelitis [8,34]. The earliest sonographic signs include periosteal thickening, which then may lead to subperiosteal fluid

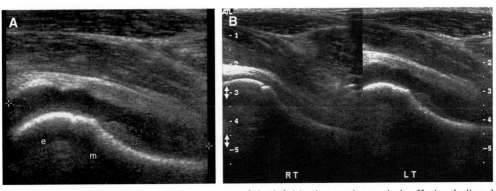

Fig. 11. Hip joint effusion. (A) Parasagittal sonogram of the left hip shows a hypoechoic effusion (calipers). (B) Comparison of normal asymptomatic right hip (RT) with the symptomatic left hip (LT) hip with effusion. e, epiphysis; m, metaphysis.

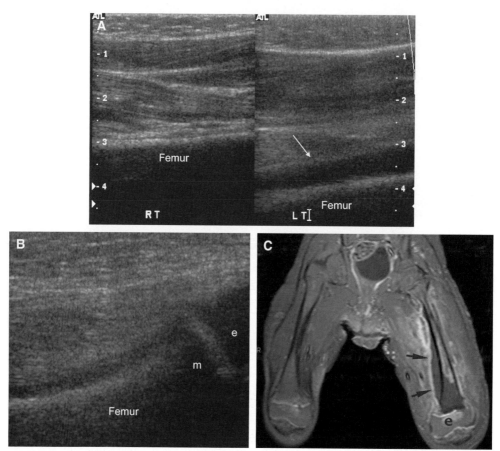

Fig. 12. Osteomyelitis and subperiosteal abscess. (*A*) Asymptomatic right (RT) posterior thigh is compared with the painful left thigh (LT), which demonstrates an anechoic layer (*arrow*) immediately adjacent to the bone (Femur), representing a subperiosteal abscess. Note the loss of definition of the muscle fibers and increased thickness of the subcutaneous tissues. (*B*) The subperiosteal collection does not extend to the epiphysis (e). (*C*) Gadolinium-enhanced T1-weighted MR imaging examination with fat saturation obtained weeks later demonstrates the subperiosteal abscess (*arrows*), which does not extend to the epiphysis (e). m, metaphysis.

(Fig. 12) and, finally, to cortical disruption [19]. The absence of sonographic findings, however, does not exclude the diagnosis. Color Doppler sonography can be helpful in follow-up examinations to evaluate the effectiveness of therapy, as the soft tissues demonstrate increased flow in advanced infection [15]. Although MR and nuclear imaging are more sensitive and used in the acute setting, metallic orthopedic hardware and prosthetic components may hamper their sensitivity rendering sonography a useful alternative.

Plain radiographs are the primary method of detection of soft tissue foreign bodies, with the exception of radiolucent objects, such as wood. Sonography provides an excellent method of localizing foreign bodies, including those that may be apparent on radiographs, to assist in precise localization [35,36]. Wooden foreign bodies as small as 2.5 mm by 1 mm are detected sonographically, with

sensitivity and specificity approaching 90% [8,19]. Foreign bodies often are echogenic with variable acoustic shadowing, a feature dependent on the object's surface rather than constituent material [11]. A foreign body with a smooth surface (such as glass or metal) has reverberations or dirty shadowing in comparison to a foreign body with an irregular surface, which has a clean shadow. The soft tissues surrounding the foreign body may demonstrate inflammation or disruption (Fig. 13). Ultrasound may provide guidance for excision, which can help to reduce time, blood loss, and tissue damage during extraction.

Low-flow vascular malformations

Although only a small percentage of vascular birthmarks requires medical evaluation, these anomalies are common entities arising in one third of the

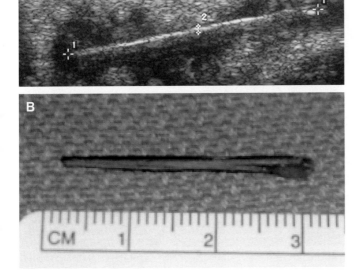

Fig. 13. Foreign body. (*A*) Sonogram of an echogenic foreign body (calipers) with surrounding hypoechoic halo. (*B*) Gross specimen of removed foreign body (wood splinter) imaged in (*A*).

population. Mulliken and Glowacki devised a classification system for these lesions [37]. The diagnosis of these lesions can be made based on clinical features, unless the lesion is deep.

Venous malformations are the most likely extremity vascular malformation to be symptomatic, producing pain and swelling. Pain may be secondary to thrombosis within the lesion or compression of adjacent structures. Leg-length discrepancy may result from accelerated growth induced by hyperemia in children who have large venous malformations. Sonographically, venous malformations appear as hypoechoic and heterogeneous masses, may contain phleboliths, and on Doppler interrogation may demonstrate low-velocity venous flow. Phleboliths are pathognomonic of venous malformations (Fig. 14) [38,39]. Sonography also enables examiners to manipulate the extremity to augment Doppler flow, by placing the extremity in a dependent position or applying compression (Fig. 15). Further assessment with MR imaging or venography may be useful for further delineation or if intervention is needed. Biopsy of any lesion is recommended if clinical and imaging features do not lead to a diagnosis.

Lymphatic malformations typically involve the face, chest, axilla, and retroperitoneum, but when they involve an extremity, localized overgrowth results. They arise from abnormal lymphatic development and may be associated with capillary or venous malformations. Lymphatic malformations can be subcategorized into microcystic and macrocystic lesions. Occasionally, these lesions increase in size and become painful secondary to hemorrhage or infection. Sonography of macrocystic lesions demonstrates large anechoic cysts with intervening septa [39]. Microcystic lymphatic malformations are nonspecific echogenic regions sonographically. Cystic lymphatic malformations can have similar imaging features with infantile fibrosarcomas and some teratomas.

Venous malformations and lymphatic malformations may be amenable to sclerotherapy using ultrasound guidance. Fluoroscopic evaluation of the venous outflow tract is evaluated before sclerotherapy of venous malformations. Surgical resection is the alternative to sclerotherapy if conservative management fails.

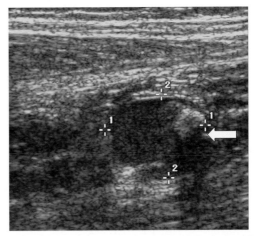

Fig. 14. Sonogram of venous malformation (calipers), containing a phlebolith with posterior acoustic shadowing (*arrow*).

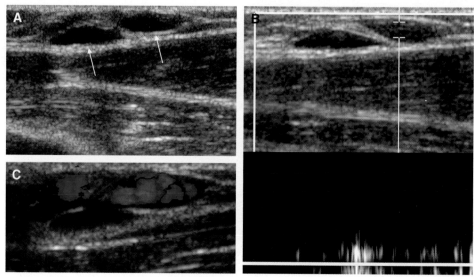

Fig. 15. Venous malformation. (*A*) Sonogram of the left upper extremity shows hypoechoic lobulations (*arrows*) representing the venous malformation. (*B*) Pulsed Doppler demonstrating low-level venous flow. (*C*) After augmentation, flow is detected with color Doppler.

Summary

As technologic improvements continue, imaging becomes increasingly more powerful and faster, having an impact on choices of modality and technique. Sonography's role in musculoskeletal imaging of pediatric patients is steadfast but evolving. The lack of radiation, ease of examination, lower cost, and dynamic nature of the sonographic examination are factors contributing to its central role in imaging in general, and its ability to demonstrate cartilaginous and soft tissue structures in patients who are skeletally immature contribute to its importance in pediatric musculoskeletal imaging in particular.

Acknowledgments

Special thanks to Diego Jaramillo, MD, MPH, for his helpful comments and cases and to Jennifer Smith, MD, for the images she contributed.

References

[1] Connell DA, Schneider-Kolsky ME, Hoving JL, et al. Longitudinal study comparing sonographic and MRI assessments of acute and healing hamstring injuries. AJR Am J Roentgenol 2004; 183:975–84.

[2] Jamadar DA, Jacobson JA, Theisen SE, et al. Sonography of the painful calf: differential considerations. AJR Am J Roentgenol 2002;179:709–16.

[3] Lee JC, Healy J. Sonography of lower limb muscle injury. AJR Am J Roentgenol 2004;182: 341–51.

[4] Koulouris G, Connell D. Hamstring muscle complex: an imaging review. Radiographics 2005; 25:571–86.

[5] Shirkhoda A, Mauro MA, Staab EV, et al. Soft-tissue hemorrhage in hemophiliac patients. Computed tomography and ultrasound study. Radiology 1983;147:811–4.

[6] Markowitz RI, Hubbard AM, Harty MP, et al. Sonography of the knee in normal and abused infants. Pediatr Radiol 1993;23:264–7.

[7] Nimkin K, Kleinman PK, Teeger S, et al. Distal humeral physeal injuries in child abuse: MR imaging and ultrasonography findings. Pediatr Radiol 1995;25:562–5.

[8] Roberts CS, Beck DJ, Heinsen J, et al. Review article diagnostic ultrasonography: applications in orthopedic surgery. Clin Orthop 2002;401: 248–64.

[9] Zieger M, Dorr U, Schulz RD. Sonography of slipped humeral epiphysis due to birth injury. Pediatr Radiol 1987;17:425–6.

[10] Ziv N, Litwin A, Katz K, et al. Definitive diagnosis of fracture-separation of the distal humeral epiphysis in neonates by ultrasonography. Pediatr Radiol 1996;26:493–6.

[11] Carr JC, Hanly S, Griffin J, et al. Sonography of the patellar tendon and adjacent structures in pediatric and adult patients. AJR Am J Roentgenol 2001;176:1535–9.

[12] Jamadar DA, Jacobson JA, Theisen SE, et al. Sonography of the painful calf: differential considerations. AJR Am J Roentgenol 2002;179: 709–16.

[13] Ward EE, Jacobson JA, Fessell DP, et al. Sonographic detection of baker's cyst. AJR Am J Roentgenol 2001;176:373–80.

[14] De Maeseneer M, Debaere C, Desprechins B, et al. Popliteal cysts in children: prevalence, appearance and associated findings at MR imaging. Pediatr Radiol 1999;29:605–9.

[15] Chao HC, Lin SJ, Huang YC, et al. Color Doppler ultrasonographic evaluation of osteomyelitis in children. J Ultrasound Med 1999;18: 729–34.

[16] Riebel TW, Nasir R, Nazarenko O. The value of sonography in the detection of osteomyelitis. Pediatr Radiol 1996;26:291–7.

[17] Sidhu PS, Rich PM. Sonographic detection and characterization of musculoskeletal and subcutaneous tissue abnormalities in sickle cell disease. Br J Radiol 1999;72:9–17.

[18] Wenaden AE, Szyszko TA, Saifuddin A. Imaging of periosteal reactions associated with focal lesions of bone. Clin Radiol 2005;60:439–56.

[19] Chau CL, Griffith JF. Musculoskeletal infections: ultrasound appearances. Clin Radiol 2005; 60:149–59.

[20] Bureau NJ, Rethy KC, Cardinal E. Musculoskeletal infections: US manifestations. Radiographics 1999;19:1585.

[21] Ruhoy MK, Tucker L, McCauley RG. Hypertrophic bursopathy of the subacromial-subdeltoid bursa in juvenile rheumatoid arthritis: sonographic appearance. Pediatr Radiol 1996;26: 353–5.

[22] Lamer S, Sebag GH. MRI and ultrasound in children with juvenile chronic arthritis. Eur J Radiol 2000;33:85–93.

[23] Buchmann RF, Jaramillo D. Imaging of articular disorders in children. Radiol Clin North Am 2004;42:151–68.

[24] Cellerini M, Salti S, Trapani S, et al. Correlation between clinical and ultrasound assessment of the knee in children with mono-articular or pauci-articular juvenile rheumatoid arthritis. Pediatr Radiol 1999;29:117–23.

[25] Newman JS, Laing TJ, McCarthy CJ, et al. Power Doppler sonography of synovitis: assessment of therapeutic response—preliminary observations. Radiology 1996;198:582–4.

[26] Doria AS, Guarniero R, Cunha FG, et al. Contrast-enhanced power Doppler sonography: assessment of revascularization flow in Legg-Calve Perthes' disease. Ultrasound Med Biol 2002; 28:171–82.

[27] Chan YL, Cheng CY, Metreweli C. Sonographic evaluation of hip effusion in children. Acta Radiol 1997;38(5):867–9.

[28] Robben SG, Lequin MH, Diepstraten AF, et al. Anterior joint capsule of the normal hip and in children with transient synovitis: US study with anatomic and histologic correlation. Radiology 1999;210:499–507.

[29] Dorr U, Zieger M, Hauke H. Ultrasonography of the painful hip. Pediatr Radiol 1988;19:36–40.

[30] Kocher MS, Zurakowski D, Kesser JR. Differentiating between septic arthritis and transient synovitis of the hip in children: an evidence-based clinical prediction algorithm. J Bone Joint Surg [Am] 1999;81:1662–70.

[31] Strouse PJ, DiPietro MA, Adler RS. Pediatric hip effusions: evaluation with power Doppler sonography. Radiology 1998;206:731–5.

[32] Robben SG, Lequin MH, Diepstraten AF, et al. Doppler sonography of the anterior ascending cervical arteries of the hip: evaluation of healthy and painful hips in children. AJR Am J Roentgenol 2000;174:1629–34.

[33] Kesteris U, Wingstrand H, Forsberg L, et al. The effect of arthrocentesis in transient synovitis of the hip in the child: a longitudinal sonographic study. J Pediatr Orthop 1996;16:24–9.

[34] Connolly LP, Connolly SA, et al. Acute hematogenous osteomyelitis of children: assessment of skeletal scintigraphy-based diagnosis in the era of MRI. J Nucl Med 2002;43:1310–6.

[35] Lin J, Jacobson JA, Fessell DP, et al. An illustrated tutorial of musculoskeletal sonography. AJR Am J Roentgenol 2000;175:1711–9.

[36] Gooding GAW, Hardiman T, Sumers M, et al. Sonography of the hand and foot in foreign body detection. J Ultrasound Med 1987;6:441–7.

[37] Mulliken JB, Glowacki J. Hemangiomas and vascular malformations in infants and children: a classification based on endothelial characteristics. Plast Reconstr Surg 1982;69:412–20.

[38] Trop I, Dubois J, Guibaud L, et al. Soft-tissue venous malformations in pediatric and young adult patients: diagnosis with Doppler US. Radiology 1999;212:841–5.

[39] Paltiel HJ, Burrows PE, Kozakewich HP, et al. Soft-tissue vascular anomalies: utility of US for diagnosis. Radiology 2000;214:747–54.

ELSEVIER
SAUNDERS

ULTRASOUND CLINICS

Ultrasound Clin 1 (2006) 509–510

Preface

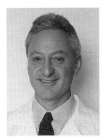
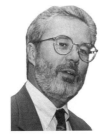

Jonathan B. Kruskal, MD, PhD
Robert A. Kane, MD
Department of Radiology
Beth Israel Deaconess Medical Center
One Deaconess Road
Boston, MA 02215, USA

E-mail addresses:
jkruskal@bidmc.harvard.edu (J.B. Kruskal)
rkane@bidmc.harvard.edu (R.A. Kane)

Jonathan B. Kruskal, MD, PhD   Robert A. Kane, MD
Guest Editors

When performed by experienced operators, intraoperative ultrasonography provides useful and often essential anatomic and staging information to the operating surgeon during complex procedures. Such applications are not limited to lesion localization and characterization, but also provide guidance for procedures, including biopsy, as well as verifying surgical margins and vascular patency.

In this issue of the *Ultrasound Clinics* a series of articles describe contemporary equipment, scanning techniques, and the more common clinical applications for intraoperative sonography in the abdomen. With many years of experience and the close collaboration of hepatobiliary and pancreatic surgeons, the authors have assembled a collection of cases that illustrate the more common abdominal pathologies likely to be encountered, as well as potential pitfalls that may occur when scanning during an open surgical procedure. Equipment requirements, including the available probe sterilization techniques, are described, coupled with specific scanning techniques relevant to each organ system being described.

Drs. Appelbaum and colleagues describe the necessary scanning techniques along with the spectrum of applications for imaging the liver. Both benign and neoplastic disorders are illustrated, as well as examples of the many clinical applications for such technology. Drs. Siewert and colleagues describe methods for imaging the intra- and extrahepatic biliary system and provide examples of the intraoperative imaging characteristics of the many infectious, inflammatory, and neoplastic disorders that involve the bile ducts. Drs. Brennan and colleagues described the intraoperative spectrum of inflammatory and neoplastic disorders of the pancreas, as well as methods required for tumor localization and staging. Finally, Drs. Ganguly and colleagues describe the equipment, sterilization methods, and scanning techniques that are necessary when performing laparoscopic ultrasonography in the upper abdomen. With advances in minimally invasive surgical applications and techniques, laparoscopic ultrasonography is being performed with increasing frequency, and this article describes the basic components of such an examination. Port insertion techniques, along with

doi:10.1016/j.cult.2006.06.002

suggested port localization sites, are illustrated, and suggested scanning techniques are provided for imaging the liver, bile ducts, and pancreas through a laparoscopic port.

Our intention in selecting these articles and authors is to illustrate the basic technical and clinical requirements for performing intraoperative sonography. Little beats clinical experience, but the information provided in these articles will provide the radiologist less experienced in intraoperative scanning methodology with sufficient knowledge to be able to provide the operating surgeon with useful information at the time of surgery.

ULTRASOUND
CLINICS

Ultrasound Clin 1 (2006) 511–520

Intraoperative Ultrasonography of the Liver: Why, When, and How?

Liat Appelbaum, MD[a,b], Jonathan B. Kruskal, MD, PhD[a,*],
Jacob Sosna, MD[a,b], Robert A. Kane, MD[a]

- Preparing for intraoperative ultrasound
  Equipment
  Scanning technique
- Relevant intraoperative anatomy
- Intraoperative specific sonographic
  technical considerations
  Surgery-specific sonographic changes
  Blind areas of the liver
  Hepatic pseudolesions
- Applications of intraoperative ultrasound
  of the liver
- *Tumor resection and metastasectomy*
- *Lesion characterization*
- *Evaluation of vessel patency*
- *Liver transplantation*
- *Guidance for procedures, including tumor
  ablation*
- *Biliary disease*
- *Clinical role of intraoperative
  ultrasonography*
- References

Intraoperative ultrasonography (IOUS) of the liver is used with increasing frequency as an adjunct to surgical planning. It provides interactive, vital, real-time information to surgeons during the procedure and has an impact on the clinical decision-making process [1,2]. IOUS of the liver has many applications, including tumor staging, metastatic surveys, guidance for metastasectomy and the various tumor ablation procedures, documentation of vessel patency, evaluation of intrahepatic biliary disease, and guidance for whole organ or split liver transplantation.

To inexperienced operators, performing an ultrasound examination in an open surgical procedure might seem daunting at first. The technique is simple to perform, however, and has a relatively short learning curve. Basic knowledge of the technical and transducer requirements, coupled with sugges-

tions for performing and interpreting the study, allows radiologists to provide useful information to surgeons during surgical procedures. This review describes transducer choice and sterilization techniques and discusses the basic requirements when preparing to enter and image in the operating room. The basic scanning techniques and relevant and variant intraoperative anatomy are illustrated along with the spectrum of unique intraoperative sonographic findings and the spectrum of clinical applications for scanning the liver in the operating room.

Preparing for intraoperative ultrasound

Equipment

Intraoperative sonography is performed best using routine mobile sonography equipment with

[a] Department of Radiology, Beth Israel Deaconess Medical Center, Harvard Medical School, Boston, MA, USA
[b] Department of Radiology, Hadassah-Hebrew University Medical Center, Jerusalem, Israel
* Corresponding author. Abdominal Imaging Section, Department of Radiology—Clinical Center 302B, Beth Israel Deaconess Medical Center, 1 Deaconess Road, Boston, MA 02215.
E-mail address: jkruskal@bidmc.harvard.edu (J.B. Kruskal).

doi:10.1016/j.cult.2006.05.007

dedicated transducers [2,3]. The liver typically is scanned with 5-MHz, side-fire, T-shaped, linear or curvilinear array transducers (Fig. 1A). The transducers should fit comfortably into the palm of a hand or between the fingers (see Fig. 1B) to allow imaging of the high dome and the right lateral segments of the liver. End-fire transducers may be used, but their role is limited because they cannot be inserted easily into the right subphrenic space. Linear or sector 7- to 7.5-MHz end-fire transducers are used typically for the gallbladder, common hepatic duct, and central intrahepatic bile ducts [4]. Transducers should be able to perform color flow and pulsed Doppler studies and have a good near-field resolution. Transducer sterilization usually is kept by using sterile condom sheaths. These should have a snug fit to avoid artifact and are essential if performing laparoscopic ultrasound. Specially designed sheaths are available for dedicated intraoperative transducers. Care should be observed when placing these near surgical retractors that may cause loose-fitting sheaths to tear. These sheaths must be long (typically approximately 1.5 m) so that the entire length of the cord can be covered.

Other sterilization options used less commonly are ethylene oxide gas sterilization, which uses a high temperature of aeration and sterilizes the probe and the supply cord. The turnaround time is 16 to 24 hours, which is slow, and several vendors claim that this may damage the skin at the transducer tip. More recently, low-temperature hydrogen peroxide gas plasma sterilization techniques have been introduced (Sterrad, Advanced Sterilization Products, Irvine, California). These systems complete an entire sterilization cycle in 2 to 3 hours, are safe to use with heat sensitive equipment, and allow sterile transducers to be used without condom sheaths. Using glutaraldehyde requires 4

hours of immersion. The authors, and most surgeons and institutions, prefer sterile condom sheaths that avoid the recognized inflammatory reaction induced by visceral contact with different techniques.

Scheduling and preoperative preparation

When preparing to perform intraoperative sonography of the liver, communication with the surgeon to establish goals and strategies is critical. Preoperative CT, MR imaging, and angiographic studies should be reviewed to maximize intraoperative interpretation. Because the time to perform these studies varies with operator experience, it is important to establish at the outset whether or not a study is a general search for metastases or being simply to help localize an impalpable lesion located deep within the liver.

To minimize the suspension of the workflow in radiology departments, the authors insist that, whenever possible, all intraoperative studies are booked ahead of time so that personnel (physicians and sonographers) and equipment can be readied and all necessary probe covers and transducers available for use. For all scheduled studies, the authors commit to being in the operating room, scrubbed and ready to scan within 15 minutes of the call from the operating room.

Operating room preparations

Radiologists must observe sterile technique; wear standard operating room gear, including gown, mask, and cap; and must scrub according to local institutional policies.

From experience, it is most helpful when a scrub nurse passes the sterile gel and sheath to a radiologist and then a sonographer is allowed to place the transducer carefully into the gel-filled sheath and to

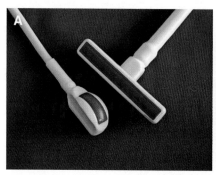 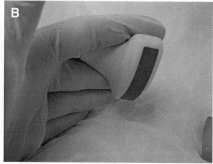

Fig. 1. Intraoperative transducers. Two, specially constructed transducers for intraoperative ultrasound of the liver are demonstrated in this example (*A*). When scanning, transducers should fit comfortably into the palm of the hand (*B*). This image shows the manner in which the intraoperative transducers should be cradled between the fingers in the palm of the hand. In this way, not only can easily exposed segments of the liver be imaged but also the transducer easily can access the more challenging locations, such as the high dome and right lateral margin.

pull the sheath carefully over the length of the cord. It is important to ensure that the covered cord is kept off the ground and away from all equipment, a task facilitated by clamping the cord to the edge of the operating field carefully. Care always should be taken to avoid sharp objects that may tear the sheath, such as surgical retractors or forceps.

Performing an ultrasound examination is an integral component of the surgical procedure and during an examination the radiologist is a full member of the operating team. For this reason, radiologists should insist on appropriate space for scanning, typically to patients' right side; should ask for the lights to be dimmed; and must ensure that the screen where images are produced is close by and easily visible.

Scanning technique

Typically, no coupling gel is required in the intraoperative setting, because the natural surface moisture of the liver is more than adequate for acoustic coupling. Bathing the field with sterile saline, however, improves acoustic coupling and helps identify lesions in the very near field that otherwise are difficult to image. To image the liver, sequential overlapping sagittal strokes should be performed with the transducer held in a transverse position, starting at the lateral-most margin of the left lateral segment 2 and extending toward the right side. In this way, the entire liver can be imaged, but this also depends on the indication for the imaging study, extent of hepatic mobilization, and incision of ligaments. It is important to make sure that the focal zone is positioned appropriately, because both near and far zones may be needed when imaging segments IV, V, and VIII. In the authors' experience, the most challenging portion to image is the high dome posterior and the blind areas of the liver. At times, it might be necessary to scan from the inferior surface of the liver, remembering to reverse or invert the images, as the probe is turned over.

Relevant intraoperative anatomy

Radiologists should be familiar with the hepatic segmental anatomy in the operating suite. It is easiest to identify the hepatic veins cranially with the transducer held in a transverse midline position angling toward the beating heart. Light pressure should be applied to the liver surface, because venous return in the retrohepatic vena cava is restricted easily in the intraoperative setting. More inferiorly, the portal veins are used for assigning segmental anatomy, best achieved by placing the transducer over segment IV b and angling toward the porta hepatis. Specific arteries that frequently

are relevant to operating surgeons include the replaced right hepatic artery arising from the superior mesenteric artery and coursing posterior to the portal vein (Fig. 2) and a replaced or accessory left hepatic artery arising from the left gastric and coursing through the ligamentum venosum (Fig. 3). Loss of the ligamentum venosum stripe may be an indicator of an isoechoic lesion adjacent to the caudate lobe of the liver (Fig. 4). Depending on the nature of a surgical procedure, the size and location of accessory hepatic veins also may need to be documented for surgeons.

Intraoperative specific sonographic technical considerations

Surgery-specific sonographic changes

For intraoperative ultrasound of the liver, certain sonographic features occur that radiologists should be aware of. The cut margin of a liver segment often is echogenic as a result of small amounts of gas that enter the parenchyma and sinusoids because of cautery or sonication, a technique commonly used for segmental resections (Fig. 5). The cut margin of partially resected tumors also may appear echogenic because of gas bubbles entering the tumor. Imaging during cauterization produces band-like artifacts (Fig. 6). Air adjacent to the vena cava, in the gallbladder fossa or in surgical packing material (Fig. 7), simulates the presence of intravenous air or produces acoustic shadowing. Cautery on the liver surface often is performed to mark subjacent lesions; this cautery produces acoustic shadowing that should be distinguished from superficial

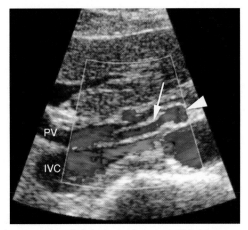

Fig. 2. Replaced right hepatic artery. This intraoperative image demonstrates a replaced right hepatic artery (*arrow*) arising from the superior mesenteric artery (*arrowhead*) and coursing between the portal vein (PV) anteriorly and the inferior vena cava (IVC) posteriorly.

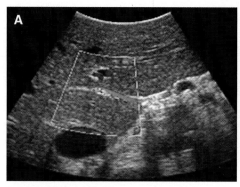 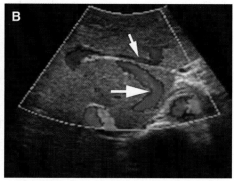

Fig. 3. Replaced left hepatic artery coursing through the ligamentum venosum. These intraoperative images demonstrate a replaced left hepatic artery coursing through the ligamentum venosum (A) that is located anterior to the caudate lobe and inferior vena cava. In (B), not only is a replaced left hepatic artery (*small arrow*) coursing through the echogenic ligamentum venosum but also a potentially significant venovenous collateral (*large arrow*) is present, the caudate lobe bridging the portal vein with the vena cava. Depiction of such vasculature is important if the surgeons are planning a resection in this anatomic region.

shadowing tumors (Fig. 8). Manual palpation on the posterior surface of the liver, frequently used to maneuver the liver for better imaging, simulates the presence of shadowing mucinous metastases (Fig. 9).

Blind areas of the liver

Certain areas of the liver are more challenging to image in the intraoperative setting. These include the high dome of the lateral right lobe that frequently requires dissection of the falciform and triangular ligaments. The posterior subdiaphragmatic bare area of the liver may be difficult to image, and surface lesions, typically hamartomas, also are difficult to identify, especially when the transducer has poor near-field resolution or the depth of field or focal zone is not altered adequately.

Hepatic pseudolesions

Focal fatty infiltration, as occurs with cirrhosis or in patients on chemotherapy, may appear quite discrete in the intraoperative setting, when image resolution is far clearer than that of the transcutaneous examination. Focal fat typically is soft and deformable by the ultrasound transducer and vessels frequently are identified coursing through the center (Fig. 10). Focal fat may occur secondary to perfusion restrictions caused by lesions. It should not cause any bulging or protrusion of the liver capsule. When focal fat is identified, it is important to image the parenchyma adjacent to the region of fat,

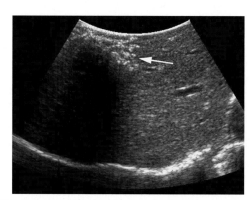

Fig. 5. Artifacts arising from sonication or cautery applied to liver surface. This intraoperative image demonstrates small echogenic bubbles (*arrow*) that have entered the liver parenchyma at the cut surface during performance of segmentectomy using a high-speed sonication device. Intrahepatic gas bubbles may be identified in hepatic segments remote from where cautery or sonication is performed and even may localize to the perisinusoidal spaces surrounding tumors.

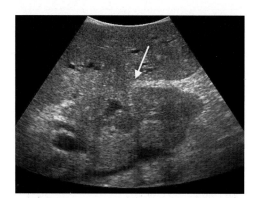

Fig. 4. Hepatic colorectal cancer metastases invading the ligamentum venosum. This intraoperative image of segments I and II of the liver demonstrates an ill-defined infiltrative colorectal cancer metastasis located primarily in the caudate lobe. The tumor has obliterated the echogenic ligamentum venosum.

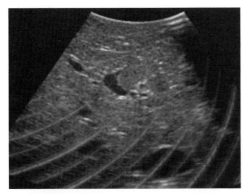

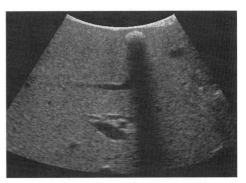

Fig. 6. Cauterization artifact during surgery. Note the linear echogenic bands radiating away from the transducer in the far field, produced when cauterization is performed while images are acquired.

Fig. 8. Cauterization artifact on liver surface. Cautery on the liver surface, performed to mark subjacent lesions producing acoustic shadowing.

because other benign entities, such as angiomyolipomas, may have a similar appearance. Focal fatty sparing typically occurs in the bare areas of the liver or abutting the porta hepatis; it may produce acoustic shadowing (Fig. 11).

Applications of intraoperative ultrasound of the liver

Tumor resection and metastasectomy

During a partial hepatectomy, surveying the entire liver for primary or metastatic lesions can be crucial. Current transducer resolution permits identification of lesions larger than 2 mm. Sensitivities of greater than 90% are documented for detection of lesions in the liver, with positive and negative predictive values of 90% and 78%, respectively [5].

Data from the authors' institution shows that IOUS routinely identifies 25% to 35% more lesions in the liver than preoperative imaging studies [6], but this number may be decreasing with improvements in resolution of other cross-sectional modalities, such as CT and MR imaging. IOUS may depict only the hyperechoic rim surrounding isodense metastases. It also is important to image lesions in two planes, because certain colorectal cancer metastases may look similar to adjacent vessels (Fig. 12).

Because hepatocellular carcinoma (frequently) and colorectal cancer metastases (rarely) can invade major vessels, it also is of immense importance to evaluate the hepatic and portal venous systems for vascular occlusion or invasion (Fig. 13) and the porta hepatis for lymphadenopathy. Documentation of the proximity of lesions to adjacent vessels depends in part on surgeons' operating technique;

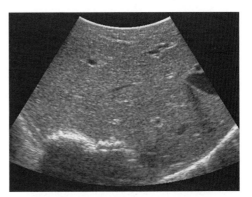

Fig. 9. Acoustic shadowing produced by manual palpation on posterior surface of the liver: This intraoperative image of the right lobe of the liver demonstrates acoustic shadowing produced by two echogenic foci in the far field. This is caused by manual pressure applied to the deep surface of the liver by the hand. Similar acoustic shadowing caused by echogenic foci may be seen with colorectal cancer metastases.

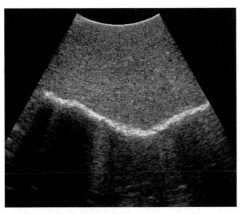

Fig. 7. Artifact produced by packing material. In the intraoperative setting, packing material frequently is used and placed around the liver surface or in the surgical bed. When imaging with ultrasound, this material usually produces acoustic shadowing obscuring structures adjacent to the liver.

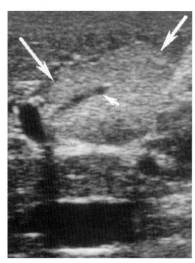

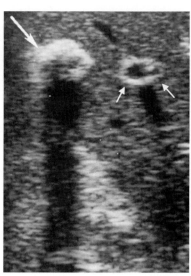

Fig. 10. Focal fatty replacement. This intraoperative image demonstrates a well-circumscribed area of increased echogenicity at the bifurcation of the main portal vein (*large arrows*). Note the small vessel coursing through the center of this region of focal fatty replacement (*small arrow*). In the intraoperative setting, areas of focal fatty replacement often are compressible.

Fig. 12. Mucinous colorectal cancer metastasis adjacent to the portal vein. This intraoperative image demonstrates acoustic shadowing produced by a small colorectal cancer metastasis (*large arrows*). Adjacent to the arrow and not producing acoustic shadowing is the portal vein (*small arrows*), which also has a rounded, echogenic appearance because of collagen within its wall.

typically margins of 1 to 2 cm are required for adequate lesion resection.

Radiologists always should keep in mind the possibility of extrahepatic disease; abnormalities in adjacent structures, such as nodes in the porta hepatis, or tumor extending into the diaphragm, right atrium, or vena cava also should be documented.

It is not uncommon to be called back to the operating room to document the extent of resection and to exclude residual tumor. For some tumors, typically located in inaccessible or challenging locations, such as the confluence of hepatic veins, it is possible that small amounts of residual tumor be identified and IOUS then can guide the additional resection.

Lesion characterization

Benign and malignant tumors frequently coexist (Fig. 14). For this reason, radiologists must be aware that metastases of similar size arising from a single primary neoplasm typically have similar sonographic appearances, whereas metastases of different sizes may have varying sonographic appearances. Therefore, if two or more lesions of similar size have differing sonographic appearances, it is likely that one set represents the neoplasm and the other set something else, such as hemangiomas.

Hemangiomas have a wide range of appearances and typically are soft and do not contain visible flow or increased flow relevant to adjacent liver parenchyma (Fig. 15). Fibrosed hemangiomas are identified by their peripheral echogenic rim.

Bull's-eye or target-appearing lesions may be seen with metastases from colon cancer, carcinoid tumors, focal nodular hyperplasia, or sarcomas (Fig. 16A,B). These may or may not contain calcifications, which are characteristically seen with mucinous gastrointestinal metastases (Fig. 17).

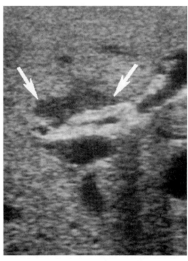

Fig. 11. Focal fatty sparing. This intraoperative image demonstrates a geographic hypoechoic region (*arrows*) abutting the right portal vein in this patient who had diffuse fatty replacement of the liver.

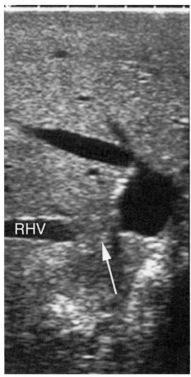

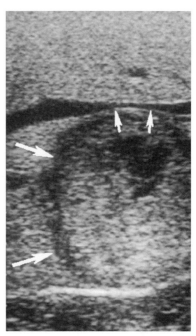

Fig. 15. Hemangioma effacing the right hepatic vein. This intraoperative image demonstrates a large echogenic hemangioma (*large arrows*) appearing to grow into the right hepatic vein (*small arrows*). The hemangioma is displacing and effacing the vein but not occluding it.

Fig. 13. Colorectal cancer metastasis invading the right hepatic vein. This intraoperative image demonstrates a colorectal cancer metastasis going into the right hepatic vein (RHV) (*arrow*) and into the vena cava. Accurate intraoperative localization of this lesion in segments VII of the liver facilitates the surgical resection.

Colon cancer metastases frequently are isoechoic to adjacent liver and, thus, may be identified by occlusion or displacement of vessels and also frequently are surrounded by an ill-defined hypoechoic rim. Fine mucinous nonshadowing calcifications may simulate hemangiomas, but metastatic tumors frequently produce shadowing, which should not occur with hemangiomas.

In selected cases, ultrasound-guided biopsy for lesions with atypical features are helpful for making the correct surgical decision.

Evaluation of vessel patency

Color flow and pulsed Doppler frequently are used to distinguish between dilated bile ducts and blood vessels (Fig. 18). When thrombus is identified in a vessel, it may be important to distinguish tumor-associated thrombus, which is avascular, from tumor thrombus, which may have an arterial waveform on pulsed Doppler evaluation. Because tumor thrombus likely renders a tumor unresectable or changes the surgical approach, it might be necessary to guide intraoperative biopsy of thrombus for diagnostic purposes. It always is important to exclude the presence of thrombus in critical areas, such as the hepatic vein confluence, the right atrium, and the intrahepatic and extrahepatic portal veins. Because benign and malignant tumors can efface vessels, it is important to distinguish between displacement and attenuation of vessels (Fig. 19), which is not a contraindication to resection, from actual invasion and occlusion of vessels.

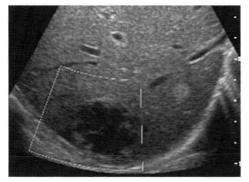

Fig. 14. Hepatocellular carcinoma and hemangioma in a 51-year-old man. This intraoperative image demonstrates a predominantly hypoechoic mass in the high dome of the liver in segment VII. Note the absence of color flow in this mass. Also note the small echogenic hemangioma located adjacent to this mass.

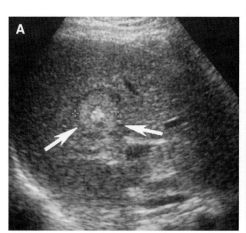

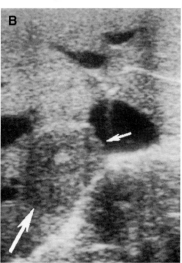

Fig. 16. Target lesions in the liver. Several different tumor types within the liver may produce target-like lesions. These are seen most commonly with colorectal cancer metastases, where the central echogenicity arises from calcification, and with carcinoid metastases (*arrows*) (*A*). Other causes of target lesions include focal nodular hyperplasia (*B*). In this example, isolated focal nodular hyperplasia (*arrows*) is extending into the inferior vena cava.

In an operative setting, Doppler ultrasound may be required to document patency and flow direction in surgically created portosystemic shunts and for characterization and surgical planning in patients who have Budd-Chiari syndrome. Depending on the nature of the surgical procedure, it might be necessary to evaluate the extrahepatic portal venous system and to guide venotomy and clot removal in some patients.

transplantation. IOUS is needed for identification of the relatively avascular resection plane 1 to 2 cm to the right of the middle hepatic vein. It also is used to document and localize the intrahepatic location of hepatic veins draining segments V and VIII and to localize and characterize accessory hepatic veins that may require separate anastomoses to be fashioned during implantation.

Liver transplantation

The major role IOUS plays in liver transplantation is during the harvesting phase in living donors when performing adult right lobe split liver

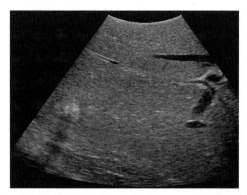

Fig. 17. Mucinous colorectal cancer metastasis. This isolated colorectal cancer metastasis contains central mucinous calcifications that are producing acoustic shadowing.

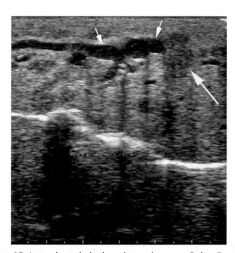

Fig. 18. Intraductal cholangiocarcinoma. Color Doppler is useful for distinguishing vessels from dilated ducts. In this case, the precise relationship between the periductal cholangiocarcinoma (*large arrow*) and the right hepatic duct (*small arrows*) is depicted, facilitating resection of the left lobe of the liver while being able to spare the right ductal system.

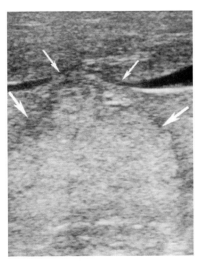

Fig. 19. Hepatic hemangiomas. In the operative setting, hemangiomas typically are soft and on Doppler studies do not demonstrate more flow than adjacent liver parenchyma. Hepatic hemangiomas vary in their appearance in the intraoperative setting. These benign tumors might demonstrate the classic, homogeneously echogenic appearance or the more atypical appearance seen with small or larger fibrosed hemangiomas. Larger hemangiomas may show easy compressibility and effacement of adjacent large vessels, such as in this example: large hemangioma effacing the right hepatic vein.

IOUS also can play a useful role in cadaveric liver transplants, where documentation of vessel patency, possible vessel injury (such as dissection), or evaluation of anastomoses may be required.

Guidance for procedures, including tumor ablation

In operative settings, IOUS may be required to guide tumor ablation treatments, such as cryoablation, ethanol ablation, microwave cautery, radiofrquency, and laser ablation. Radiologists should be familiar with the sonographic changes that occur during instillation or ablation [1,7]. Because the treatment may produce acoustic shadowing, for monitoring of needle or electrode location and efficacy of treatment, it frequently is necessary to image the liver from the contralateral sides to that of probe insertion.

Biliary disease

Although IOUS is used to image extrahepatic bile duct abnormalities, including retained stones, and to locate cystic duct insertion sites, many intrahepatic biliary abnormalities occur and can be evaluated thoroughly with ultrasound [4]. IOUS is used to define ductal anatomy and to locate the site of confluence of the right and left hepatic ducts in

patients who have resectable cholangiocarcinoma, to locate and characterize bile duct strictures, and to define the extent of segmental involvement in patients who have chronic inflammatory changes, Caroli's disease, and recurrent pyogenic cholangiohepatitis. Color Doppler is used to distinguish dilated ducts from vessels (Fig. 18) and to distinguish intrabiliary sludge from tumor. Chronic inflammatory changes of the gallbladder and bile ducts are difficult to distinguish from malignancies, but ultrasound plays a particularly useful role in guiding resection. Most commonly, however, IOUS is used to exclude metastases when patients are undergoing trisegmental resections for cholangiocarcinoma.

Clinical role of intraoperative ultrasonography

It was shown that IOUS can change the clinical management in up to 50% of patients undergoing hepatic resection for malignancy [8,9–12]. Even when IOUS has not modified surgical management [12], however, it has correctly changed the stage of the disease and consequently of postoperative treatment in 11% of patients [13]. In a substantial proportion of patients undergoing hepatic resection, IOUS provides additional specificity in the evaluation of liver lesions [14]. In a prospective evaluation, the authors show that IOUS showed 25% to 35% additional lesions compared with preoperative ultrasound, CT, and angiography. More importantly, 40% of the lesions demonstrated by IOUS were neither visible nor palpable at surgery [6]. Although IOUS helps to determine the anatomic location of metastases, its adjunctive use in patients screened preoperatively by fluorodeoxyglucose positron emission tomography may have limited impact on treatment selection [15].

The performance and usefulness of IOUS in patients who have colorectal cancer metastases may depend on operator experience and the extent of underlying liver disease. Although Schmidt and colleagues [16] show a sensitivity and specificity of 98% of 95%, respectively, for detection of colorectal cancer metastases, Leen and coworkers [17] show that IOUS is relatively insensitive in the detection of occult colorectal liver metastases. A study from the authors' institution shows that the small increment in detection of occult metastases does not warrant its use in all patients who have colorectal cancer [18]. Selective use in patients who have T3 or T4 lesions or recurrent cancers increases the incremental gain in detection to the extent that the authors suggest that the observed frequency of occult metastases in patients who have T3 tumors (12.5%) is sufficient to have an impact on the results of adjuvant chemotherapy trials [18]. Other investigators show that IOUS supplies additional information in up to 38% of operations [8].

The technical performance of preoperative hepatic imaging has improved considerably in recent years. In a recent performance comparison between IOUS and contrast-enhanced MR, the sensitivities of MR imaging and IOUS for liver lesion depiction were 86.7% and 94.3%, respectively [19]. Bloed and coworkers [20] show that despite preoperative triphasic CT imaging, IOUS still provided additional useful information in 50% of their patients, resulting in a change in surgical procedure in 15%.

In summary, IOUS of the liver is a useful surgical adjunct and provides diagnostic and staging information to surgeons during operative procedures. The real-time information provided to surgeons may result in an alteration in planned surgical approach. The technique is simple to perform and has a relatively short learning curve.

References

[1] Kruskal JB, Kane RA. Intraoperative ultrasonography of the liver. Crit Rev Diagn Imaging 1995; 36:175–226.

[2] Silas AM, Kruskal JB, Kane RA. Intraoperative ultrasound. Radiol Clin North Am 2001;39:429–48.

[3] Reading CC. Intraoperative sonography. Abdomen Imaging 1996;21:21–9.

[4] Kruskal JB, Kane RA. Intraoperative sonography of the biliary system. AJR Am J Roentgenol 2001;177:395–403.

[5] Guimaraes CM, Correia MM, Baldisserotto M, et al. Intraoperative ultrasonography of the liver in patients with abdominal tumors: a new approach. J Ultrasound Med 2004;23:1549–55.

[6] Clarke MP, Kane RA, Steele G Jr, et al. Prospective comparison of preoperative imaging and intraoperative ultrasonography in the detection of liver tumors. Surgery 1989;106:849–55.

[7] Solbiati L, Ierace T, Tonolini M, et al. Guidance and monitoring of radiofrequency liver tumor ablation with contrast-enhanced ultrasound. Eur J Radiol 2004;51(Suppl):S19–23.

[8] Boutkan H, Luth W, Meyer S, et al. The impact of intraoperative ultrasonography of the liver on the surgical strategy of patients with gastrointestinal malignancies and hepatic metastases. Eur J Surg Oncol 1992;18:342–6.

[9] Kane RA, Hughes LA, Cua EJ, et al. The impact of intraoperative ultrasonography on surgery for liver neoplasms. J Ultrasound Med 1994;13:1–6.

[10] Solomon MJ, Stephen MS, Gallinger S, et al. Does intraoperative hepatic ultrasonography change surgical decision making during liver resection? Am J Surg 1994;168:307–10.

[11] Cervone A, Sardi A, Conaway GL. Intraoperative ultrasound (IOUS) is essential in the management of metastatic colorectal liver lesions. Am Surg 2000;66:611–5.

[12] Conlon R, Jacobs M, Dasgupta D, et al. The value of intraoperative ultrasound during hepatic resection compared with improved preoperative magnetic resonance imaging. Eur J Ultrasound 2003;16:211–6.

[13] Paul MA, Mulder LS, Cuesta MA, et al. Impact of intraoperative ultrasonography on treatment strategy for colorectal cancer. Br J Surg 1994; 81:1660–3.

[14] Haider MA, Leonhardt C, Hanna SS, et al. The role of intraoperative ultrasonography in planning the resection of hepatic neoplasms. Can Assoc Radiol J 1995;46:98–104.

[15] Rydzewski B, Dehdashti F, Gordon BA, et al. Usefulness of intraoperative sonography for revealing hepatic metastases from colorectal cancer in patients selected for surgery after undergoing FDG PET. AJR Am J Roentgenol 2002;178:353–8.

[16] Schmidt J, Strotzer M, Fraunhofer S, et al. Intraoperative ultrasonography versus helical computed tomography and computed tomography with arterioportography in diagnosing colorectal liver metastases: lesion-by-lesion analysis. World J Surg 2000;24:43–7.

[17] Leen E, Angerson WJ, O'Gorman P, et al. Intraoperative ultrasound in colorectal cancer patients undergoing apparently curative surgery: correlation with two year follow-up. Clin Radiol 1996;51:157–9.

[18] Stone MD, Kane R, Bothe A Jr, et al. Intraoperative ultrasound imaging of the liver at the time of colorectal cancer resection. Arch Surg 1994; 129:431–5.

[19] Sahani DV, Kalva SP, Tanabe KK, et al. Intraoperative US in patients undergoing surgery for liver neoplasms: comparison with MR imaging. Radiology 2004;232:810–4.

[20] Bloed W, van Leeuwen MS, Borel et al. Role of intraoperative ultrasound of the liver with improved preoperative hepatic imaging. Eur J Surg 2000;166:691–5.

ELSEVIER
SAUNDERS

ULTRASOUND CLINICS

Ultrasound Clin 1 (2006) 521–531

Intraoperative Sonography of the Biliary System

Bettina Siewert, MD[a,b,]*, Jonathan B. Kruskal, MD, PhD[a,b],
Robert A. Kane, MD, FACR[a,b]

- Transducer choice and options
- Transducer sterilization
- Intraoperative scanning technique
- Relevant surgical anatomy of biliary system

- Clinical applications
  - *Gallbladder diseases*
  - *Diseases of the bile ducts*
- Summary
- References

Intraoperative sonography (IOUS) of the biliary system originally was restricted to examination of the gallbladder and calculus disease, where it has been demonstrated to be more cost effective and time efficient than intraoperative cholangiography during laparoscopic cholecystectomy [1]. It is increasingly important, however, in all aspects of biliary surgery [2]. Intraoperative sonography allows accurate segmental anatomic localization of bile duct lesions, which is helpful in surgical planning. When characterization of bile duct lesions is possible and benign disease can be differentiated from malignant disease, this has major impact on surgical technique and extent of resection. In the case of malignant disease, sonography can be used for staging of neoplasms and to evaluate for metastatic disease to the liver. Several investigators point out that a considerable learning curve exists for this technique [3] and that for the evaluation of bile duct anatomy and stones alone, examiners have to have performed at least 10 examinations [1].

Transducer choice and options

For intraoperative sonography of the bile ducts during laparotomy, 7.5- or 10.0-MHz linear array or convex array transducers are preferable [4,5]. Sector probes are used when a larger field of view is warranted, whereas linear array probes improve near-field definition. For examination of the intrahepatic bile ducts, 5-MHz, side-fire, T-shaped probes are preferred. These also can be used if the extrahepatic bile ducts are imaged through the liver parenchyma. For imaging of deeper structures, such as the distal common bile duct and common hepatic duct, smaller end-fire probes are used. All transducers have to be equipped with pulsed Doppler and color flow ability, which is critical in differentiating bile ducts from vessels.

For laparoscopic procedures, sonography is performed with a flexible tip 5- to 7.5-MHz transducer. The intrahepatic biliary tree is visualized best with the transducer advanced through the right upper quadrant or a left paramedian port, as the falciform

[a] Department of Radiology, Beth Israel Deaconess Medical Center, Boston, MA, USA
[b] Harvard Medical School, Boston, MA, USA
* Corresponding author. Department of Radiology, Beth Israel Deaconess Medical Center, 1 Deaconess Road, Boston, MA 00215.
E-mail address: bsiewert@bidmc.harvard.edu (B. Siewert).

1556-858X/06/$ – see front matter © 2006 Elsevier Inc. All rights reserved.
ultrasound.theclinics.com

doi:10.1016/j.cult.2006.05.008

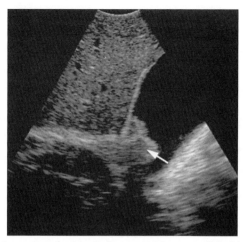

Fig. 1. Tumefactive sludge presenting as gallbladder mass of heterogeneous echotexture (*arrow*) and absent color flow. The mass extends into the cystic duct. Preoperative diagnosis of gallbladder carcinoma was suspected. Surgical resection was limited as findings were consistent with benign disease.

ligament limits transducer mobility over the liver surface [6]. Examination of the extrahepatic bile ducts is performed through the umbilical or left paramedian ports.

Transducer sterilization

Effective transducer sterility can be achieved by gas sterilization or with the use of sterile cover sheaths. At the authors' institution, ethylene oxide gas sterilization is performed, because it does not leave any harmful residue on the probe, the risk for a torn probe cover can be avoided, and no problems have been experienced with this technique. The high temperatures of aeration after gas exposure, however, may damage the delicate outer coating of the transducer head and, therefore, this technique is not approved by some manufacturers. The gas sterilization process takes approximately 24 hours and, thus, each probe can be used only once a day. Advanced planning for surgical procedures requiring intraoperative sonography, therefore, is required. Cover sheaths is a simpler method of achieving sterility during the surgical procedure. Covers need to be designed

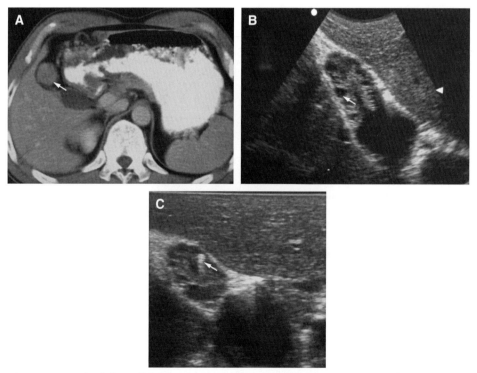

Fig. 2. Adenomyomatosis of the gallbladder. (*A*) CT examination demonstrates a mass in the gallbladder fundus (*arrow*). (*B*) Intraoperative ultrasound demonstrates small cystic spaces in the gallbladder wall representing Rokitansky-Aschoff sinuses (*arrow*), a characteristic finding in adenomyomatosis. (*C*) Crystal in Rokitansky-Aschoff sinus causing ringdown artifact (*arrow*), another typical finding in adenomyomatosis. Surgical resection thus could be limited to cholecystectomy.

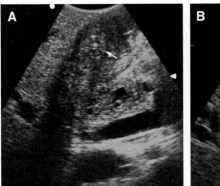
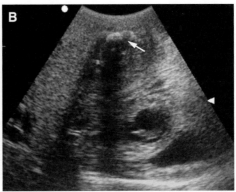

Fig. 3. Xanthogranulomatous cholecystitis. (*A*) A massive circumferential wall thickening of the gallbladder (*arrow*) is noted in the presence of (*B*) shadowing gallstones (*arrow*) and sludge. Intraoperative biopsy was performed using sonographic guidance and confirmed inflammatory changes. Surgery could be limited to cholecystectomy.

specifically for a given transducer head, however, to accomplish a snug fit and, thus, minimize artifact. In addition, tightly fitting covers are less likely to be damaged by surgical instruments and retractors.

Intraoperative scanning technique

During open laparotomy, examination of the intrahepatic and most of the extrahepatic biliary tree is performed by placing the transducer directly onto the moist anterior surface of the liver. The extrahepatic bile ducts may be imaged through the head of the pancreas or the liver parenchyma. Because of near-field limitations, visualization of the

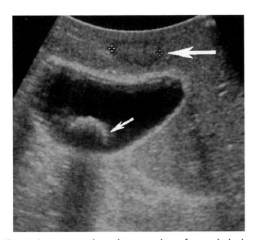

Fig. 4. Intraoperative ultrasound performed during cholecystectomy (for cholelithiasis) (*small arrow*) was performed for evaluation of choledocholithiasis demonstrating incidental finding of a liver lesion with a hypoechoic rim (*large arrow*). Ultrasound-guided biopsy was performed intraoperatively and confirmed metastatic disease from an unknown primary.

extrahepatic ducts may be improved by instillation of warmed, sterile saline into the abdominal cavity. If necessary, imaging of the common bile duct in the head of the pancreas can be improved by surgical mobilization of the duodenal C-sweep. This, however, is rarely, if ever, performed. Color Doppler imaging frequently is necessary for distinguishing dilated bile ducts from adjacent portal vein branches in the liver.

Examination of the gallbladder is performed through the liver when possible. This approach avoids near-field artifact and minimizes the chance of missing lesions in the near field. Color Doppler imaging is helpful in confirming the presence of tumefactive sludge by demonstrating the absence of color flow in what often appears as an intraluminal mass.

Relevant surgical anatomy of biliary system

Radiologists have to be familiar with normal and variant bile duct anatomy, as it is important for localizing disease and surgical planning. The presence of percutaneous biliary catheters, if inserted before surgery to decompress dilated ducts, often facilitates localization of intra- and extrahepatic ducts. Normal caliber intrahepatic bile ducts easily are visible toward the center of the liver. Peripheral intrahepatic ducts are difficult to discern, unless they are dilated. Occasionally, however, isolated peripheral branches may be visualized, particularly in the left lobe of the liver. When guiding hepatic incisions during right lobe of liver harvesting before implantation, it is important to be aware of aberrant right hepatic ducts that cross to enter into the left hepatic duct. During biliary and pancreatic resections, it may be necessary to document the precise site of insertion of the cystic duct where it joins the common hepatic duct to form the common bile duct. The

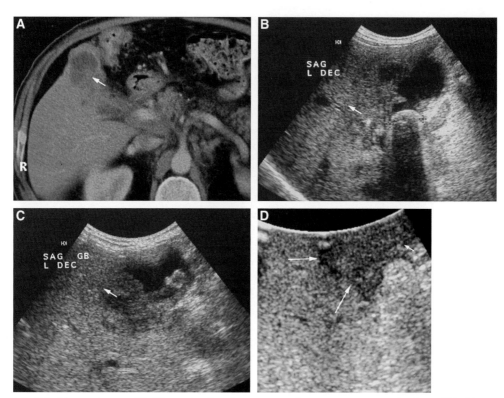

Fig. 5. Gallbladder carcinoma. (*A*) CT examination demonstrates heterogeneous mass in the gallbladder; extension of the mass into the liver parenchyma is difficult to delineate. (*B,C*) Intraoperative ultrasound confirms heterogeneous mass in the gallbladder with extension into the liver (*arrow*). (*D*) Intraoperative ultrasound shows a small superficial liver lesion (*arrows*) not identified on CT imaging. Ultrasound-guided biopsy was performed intraoperatively and confirmed metastatic disease.

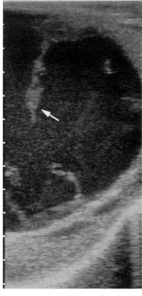

Fig. 6. Hemorrhagic cyst. Complex cyst with a thin wall and mobile septations (*arrow*) with absence of color flow within the septations. Mobile septations and absence of color flow are consistent with a diagnosis of hemorrhage into a simple cyst.

cystic duct originates close to the transverse Heister's valves of the gallbladder and can be followed to its insertion into the common bile duct. Depending on the nature of the anticipated surgical procedure, the precise site of insertion may be important to document, because this may alter the planned operation.

Clinical applications

Gallbladder diseases

Benign gallbladder diseases

Intraoperative sonography can be helpful in distinguishing benign from malignant processes and, thus, influence surgical approach. Tumefactive sludge demonstrates a characteristic echotexture, is easily compressible, and demonstrates no color flow (Fig. 1). Adenomyomatosis of the gallbladder can occur as a focal mass in the fundus but has a characteristic sonographic appearance with small crystal-containing anechoic cystic lesions in the gallbladder wall, representing Rokitansky-Aschoff sinuses (Fig. 2). Xanthogranulomatous cholecystitis demonstrates massive circumferential thickening

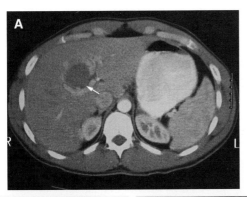

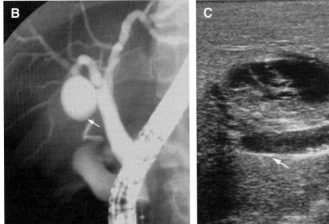

Fig. 7. Intrahepatic choledochal cyst. (*A*) CT examination demonstrates a cystic intrahepatic lesion (*arrow*). (*B*) Endoscopic retrograde cholangiopancreatography confirms connection with the bile duct and, thus, presence of a choledochal cyst (*arrow*). (*C*) Intraoperative ultrasound demonstrates a cystic mass with internal septations and defines adjacent vasculature (*arrow*).

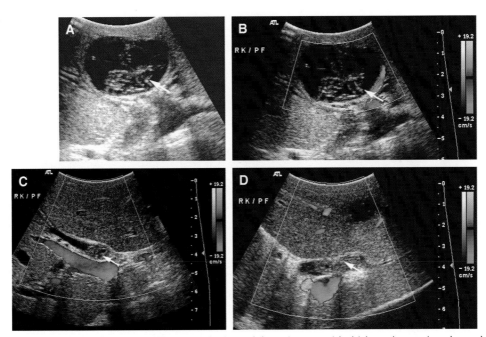

Fig. 8. Biliary cystadenoma extending into the bile ducts. (*A*) Cystic mass with thickened septations (*arrow*) demonstrates color flow in septations (*arrow*) (*B*). (*C*) Echogenic material is seen extending into the right hepatic duct (*arrow*). (*D*) Color flow within the echogenic material confirms that this represents soft tissue (*arrow*). A left hemihepatectomy was performed as the soft tissue in the right hepatic duct easily could be removed.

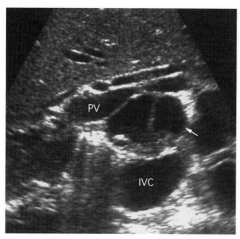

Fig. 9. Extrahepatic biliary cystadenoma. On intraoperative ultrasound, there is a small cystic mass (*arrow*) in the porta hepatis. Sonography identifies adjacent vascular structures, such as portal vein (PV) and inferior vena cava (IVC), and helps guide surgical resection.

of the gallbladder wall (Fig. 3). Stones and sludge may be seen in the gallbladder lumen. Although the circumferential nature of the gallbladder wall thickening favors an inflammatory process, ultimately, diffuse involvement with gallbladder carcinoma cannot be excluded and intraoperative biopsy may be necessary to confirm the diagnosis. Because inflammatory processes, such as in chronic cholecystitis, can extend into the cystic and common bile duct, examination of these structures is necessary for surgical planning. During laparoscopic cholecystectomy, laparoscopic sonography can be used to evaluate the bile ducts for residual stones (Fig. 4) and to document the site of cystic duct insertion [8]. Variations of the hepatic artery anatomy are detected in 22% of these patients [9]. In patients undergoing gastric bypass surgery, intraoperative sonography is demonstrated to identify gallbladder disease in 17% of patients who had no palpable abnormalities during surgery. These

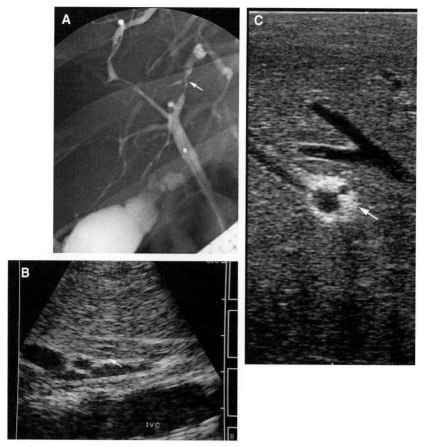

Fig. 10. Primary sclerosing cholangitis. Endoscopic retrograde cholangiopancreatography demonstrates segmental narrowing (*arrow*) and dilatation of intrahepatic bile ducts. (*B*) Intraoperative sonography shows circumferential thickening (*arrow*) of the wall of the common hepatic duct. Note the narrow central lumen. (*C*) Bile duct walls can be markedly hyperechoic (*arrow*). Note adjacent portal vein.

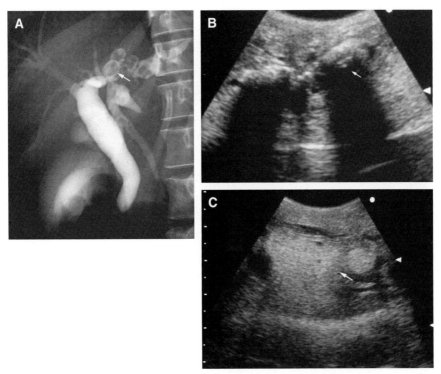

Fig. 11. Recurrent cholangiohepatitis. (*A*) Cholangiogram demonstrates dilated segmental bile ducts in the left lateral lobe with multiple filling defects (*arrow*) from stones. (*B*) Intraoperative sonogram confirms multiple shadowing stones in the left lateral segment (*arrow*). (*C*) Echogenic nonshadowing stones (*arrow*) are seen in the medial segments ducts. This finding changed the surgical procedure, requiring a left hemihepatectomy instead of the scheduled lateral segmentectomy.

patients typically undergo cholecystectomy at the time of bariatric surgery [10].

Malignant diseases of the gallbladder

In the intraoperative setting, sonography may be required to document extension of hepatic tumors into the gallbladder or vice versa (Fig. 5). The extent of invasion into the liver bed is difficult for surgeons to determine by inspection and palpation and can be depicted well using intraoperative sonography [11]. An aggressive resection of all contiguous tumor that has invaded the liver is essential to achieve any long-term survival or surgical cure, and intraoperative sonography is able to provide an accurate depiction of the precise location and depth of intrahepatic invasion. Certain malignancies have a propensity to involve the gallbladder, such as melanoma, and biliary involvement may be identified in the operative setting. Gallbladder carcinoma may present as a focal mural-based intraluminal mass with increased color flow. Intraoperative sonography outlines tumor margins and depth of infiltration. Scanning of the liver is performed to rule out hepatic metastases. If stones are present in the

gallbladder, the common bile duct can be investigated for the retained stones at the same time. During cholecystectomy for gallbladder carcinoma, intraoperative sonography identifies the depth of invasion and defines resection margins if the tumor infiltrates the liver parenchyma. Other entities may simulate a gallbladder malignancy, including xanthogranulomatous cholecystitis (Fig. 3) and segmental adenomyomatosis (Fig. 2).

Diseases of the bile ducts

Cystic masses

Simple cysts of the biliary system meet surgical criteria for removal if they become symptomatic (often through hemorrhage [Fig. 6]), if they cannot be distinguished confidently from biliary cystadenomas or cystadenocarcinomas, or if a cystic lesion is considered to be a choledochal cyst (Fig. 7) that needs to be removed because of risk for developing cholangiocarcinoma. In choledochal cysts, communication with the bile ducts can be documented to limit extent of resection. If there is concern for cholangiocarcinoma developing in a choledochal cyst, intraoperative sonography can be used to identify

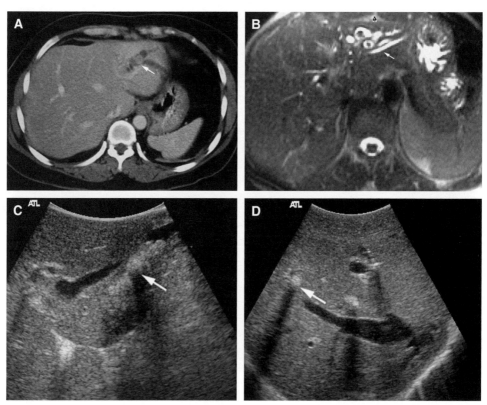

Fig. 12. Caroli's disease. (*A*) CT examination demonstrates dilated ducts in the lateral segment of the liver (*arrow*). (*B*) Axial T2-weighted MR imaging confirmed ductal dilatation (*arrow*) and revealed debris within the bile ducts. (*C*) The extent of ductal involvement is best appreciated on intraoperative sonogram, where debris (*arrow*) was noted in the known location in the left lobe; however, examination of the right lobe confirmed debris scattered throughout the right lobe (arrow) (*D*). Resection thus was limited to the left lobe.

involvement of the adjacent bile ducts (Fig. 8) or gallbladder, because the entire biliary system is at risk for cholangiocarcinoma and sonography also can be used to search for intrahepatic metastases.

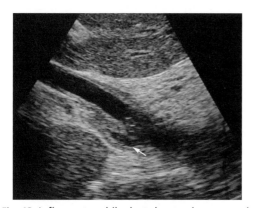

Fig. 13. Inflammatory bile duct changes in pancreatic adenocarcinoma. Intraoperative sonogram demonstrates circumferential bile duct wall thickening of the common bile duct, common hepatic duct, and cystic duct (*arrow*) resulting from chronic inflammation.

Complex cystic masses need to undergo surgery if benignity cannot be established by imaging. A thin cyst wall with few thin septations and lack of color flow within septations favors a benign etiology and, thus, more limited resection may be feasible. Differentiation from a malignant neoplasm may be difficult particularly in lesions that are multiseptated or that have undergone hemorrhage or infection, as their imaging appearance can be complex. Intraoperative sonography localizes a lesion within a segment accurately and identifies the relationship of a cyst to vascular structures in the vicinity (Fig. 9). Color flow imaging may be helpful, particularly demonstrating adjacent vascular structures. The proximity of the cyst to the surface of the liver can be assessed. If biopsy of complex cystic masses is warranted, intraoperative sonography is helpful in identifying a suitable location for biopsy.

Infectious and inflammatory disorders of the bile ducts

Among the diseases that affect the bile ducts and may require surgical intervention are sclerosing cholangitis, Caroli's disease, recurrent pyogenic

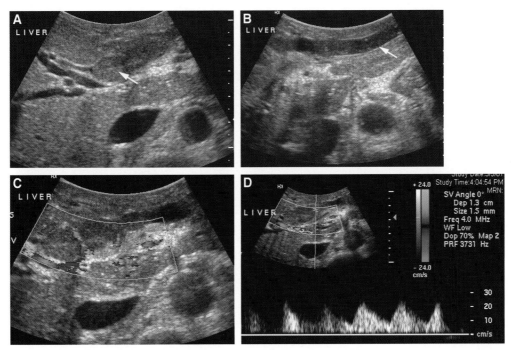

Fig. 14. Cholangiocarcinoma. (*A*) Intraoperative sonogram reveals soft tissue mass (*arrow*) expanding the left hepatic duct. (*B*) Image obtained cranial to (*A*) demonstrates dilated duct (*arrow*) proximal to the lesion. (*C*) Color examination demonstrates flow within the soft tissue. (*D*) Doppler examination confirms arterial waveform consistent with tumor infiltration.

cholangiohepatitis, and cholangiocarcinoma. Primary sclerosing cholangitis may cause marked circumferential wall thickening of the bile ducts, often without any dilatation of the duct lumen (Fig. 10). The intrahepatic duct walls may be hyperechoic and minimal segmental intrahepatic ductal dilatation may be identified. In addition, small

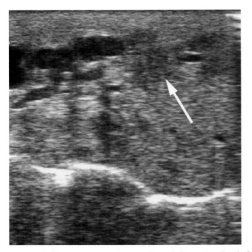

Fig. 15. Cholangiocarcinoma. Dilated ducts in the left lobe resulting from small obstructing hypoechoic mass (*arrow*) extending into the liver parenchyma.

intrahepatic duct stones occasionally may be seen. In patients who have sclerosing cholangitis, other hepatic findings that may occur include solitary or multiple abscesses or cholangiocarcinoma. Recurrent pyogenic cholangiohepatitis produces marked dilatation of bile ducts in a segmental or lobar distribution. Stones or sludge can be seen in these dilated ducts and may be the only sign of segmental involvement in the absence of ductal dilatation [7]. Intraductal stones and sludge frequently do not produce much acoustic shadowing and appear as homogeneous echogenic material within a dilated duct (Fig. 11). Caroli's disease can be limited to individual hepatic segments and may appear as isolated dilated ducts containing stones, sludge (Fig. 12), or even gas. Recurrent pyogenic cholangiohepatitis and Caroli's disease may be difficult to distinguish from each other by imaging alone. In an intraoperative setting, chronic cholecystitis and diseases involving the head of the pancreas also may produce changes in the extrahepatic bile ducts (Fig. 13). These changes, however, often are focal and associated with dilatation of the more proximal ducts.

Malignant diseases of the bile ducts

It is important to emphasize that chronic inflammatory diseases of the bile ducts, especially primary sclerosing cholangitis, and cholangiocarcinoma

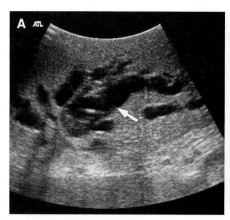 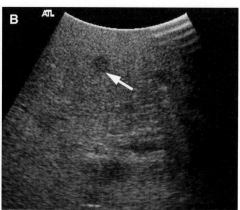

Fig. 16. Cholangiocarcinoma. (*A*) Extensive biliary ductal dilatation (*arrow*) without an obstructing mass is noted. (*B*) Hypoechoic liver lesion (*arrow*) not identified on preoperative imaging studies was biopsied intraoperatively using sonographic guidance. This revealed metastatic disease.

may be indistinguishable in the operative setting. Both are likely to produce duct wall thickening and dilatation of proximal ducts. A subtle hyperechoic mass may be visible in the liver contiguous to the dilated ducts. Although cholangiocarcinoma most commonly produces circumferential duct wall thickening, occasionally, cholangiocarcinoma may present as an intraluminal mass within a dilated bile duct (Fig. 14) that can be identified at the site of obstruction. More commonly, however, an area of focal wall thickening with or without extra

luminal extension may be noted (Fig. 15). Doppler examination may establish flow within the tissue and help differentiation from sludge (Fig. 14).

When patients are undergoing a lobar resection, intraoperative sonography is important especially for identifying the location of the confluence of the left and right hepatic ducts. The ability to exclude involvement of the contralateral hepatic ducts may limit the extent of surgical resection (Fig. 14). This is important particularly as the extent of wall thickening of bile ducts may be underappreciated on preoperative imaging modalities. Examination of the entire biliary tree also is necessary as additional findings, such as stones, in other segments may lead to more extensive resection.

Intraoperative sonography of the liver is an important part of the staging examination to rule out hepatic metastases. This can identify occult disease not identifiable on inspection or palpation of the liver during surgery and not depicted on prior imaging evaluation because of small lesion size. If liver lesions are identified at the time of surgery, ultrasound can assist in lesion characterization by identifying them as simple cysts or guiding intraoperative biopsy of small, solid, nonpalpable liver lesions (Figs. 4, 16).

Imaging of the extrahepatic bile ducts may be necessary in patients undergoing resections of pancreatic head masses. During resection for pancreatic carcinoma, sonographic examination of the bile ducts can establish the extent of involvement and, thus, influence the decision regarding which type of biliary anastomoses needs to be performed. A cholecystojejunal anastomosis, the simpler surgical procedure, is feasible when there is no ductal involvement superior to the cystic duct insertion site (Fig. 17). More proximal involvement may require a hepaticojejunal anastomosis. Staging of tumors

Fig. 17. Involvement of the common bile duct in a patient who had pancreatic carcinoma. There is thickening of the common bile duct (*thick arrow*) extending inferior to the insertion of the cystic duct (*thin arrow*). Cholecystojejunal anastomosis thus could be performed.

should include not only a search for local spread and nodal involvement but also scanning to identify any liver metastases.

Summary

Intraoperative ultrasonography can serve as a useful adjunct to surgical procedures involving the intra- and extrahepatic biliary system. The technique is used to localize and characterize disease entities, to facilitate surgical planning and tumor staging, and to guide surgeons when performing resections. With rapid advances being made in the spectrum of minimally invasive procedures, an increased demand is anticipated for intraoperative sonography when patients are undergoing resections of complex biliary disorders.

References

[1] Falcone RA, Fegelman EJ, Nussbaum MS, et al. A prospective comparison of laparoscopic ultrasound vs intraoperative cholangiogram during laparoscopic cholecystectomy. Surg Endosc 1999;13:784–8.

[2] Gigot JF, Kestens PJ. The role of intraoperative ultrasound in biliary surgery: results and critical evaluation in cholelithiasis and biliary cancer. In: Gozzetti G, Mazziotti A, Bolondi L, et al, editors. Intraoperative ultrasonography in hepato-biliary and pancreatic surgery. Dordrect (The Netherlands): Kluwer Academic Publishers; 1989. p. 97–133.

[3] Catheline JM, Turner R, Rizk N, et al. Evaluation of the biliary tree during laparoscopic ultrasound versus intraoperative cholangiography: a prospective study of 150 cases. Surg Laparosc Endosc 1998;8:85–91.

[4] Kruskal JB, Kane RA. Intraoperative ultrasonography of the liver. Crit Rev Diagn Imaging 1995; 36:175–226.

[5] Reading CC. Intraoperative sonography. Abdom Imaging 1996;21:21–9.

[6] Glaser KS, Tschmelitsch J, Klinger A, et al. Is there a role for laparoscopic ultrasonography (LUS)? Surg Laparosc Endosc 1995;5:370–5.

[7] Kruskal JB, Kane RA. Intraoperative sonography of the biliary system. AJR Am J Roentgenol 2001;177:395–4003.

[8] Merhar GL. Intraoperative biliary ultrasound. In: Kane RA, editor. Intraoperative, laparoscopic, and endoluminal ultrasound. Philadelphia: Churchill Livingstone; 1999. p. 75–89.

[9] Rothlin MA, Schlumpf R, Largiader F. Laparoscopic sonography. An alternative to routine intraoperative cholangiography? Arch Surg 1994; 129:694–700.

[10] Herbst CA, Mittelsteadt CA, Staab EV, et al. Intraoperative ultrasonography evaluation of the gallbladder in morbidly obese patients. Ann Surg 1984;200:691–2.

[11] Azuma T, Yoshikawa T, Araida T, et al. Intraoperative evaluation of the depth of invasion of gallbladder cancer. Am J Surg 1999;178:381–4.

ELSEVIER
SAUNDERS

ULTRASOUND
CLINICS

Ultrasound Clin 1 (2006) 533–545

Intraoperative Ultrasound of the Pancreas

Darren D. Brennan, MD*, Jonathan B. Kruskal, MD, PhD,
Robert A. Kane, MD, FACR

Intraoperative ultrasound (IOUS) of the pancreas first was described in 1980 by Lane and Glazer [1] and has since established itself as one of the major applications of this technology. Used initially as a diagnostic tool, its versatility has led to its adaptation for several intraoperative interventions, including biopsy, drainage, ablation, and duct cannulation. Although there have been many advances in cross-sectional technologies since its inception, the unparalleled spatial and contrast resolution of IOUS still makes it indispensable to pancreatic surgeons. It can be used to define lesions, characterize them, and delineate their anatomic relationships and to evaluate the pancreatic and biliary ductal system. In defining disease extent, it influences choice of surgical procedure. With a skilled operator and good working relationship with surgical colleagues, radiologists can offer an important contribution to patient management without unduly compromising work flow in radiology departments.

Transducer requirements

Choice of transducer

IOUS of the pancreas is performed best with an end-fire transducer [2], as the side-fire transducers used in hepatic imaging are unsuited to the contours of the gland. The authors typically bring linear and sector probes to the operating suite (Fig. 1); the actual transducer used depends on the clinical situation. The typical frequencies used are 7.5 to 10 MHz, although linear high-resolution transducers of up to 12.5 MHz are applied to good effect in some circumstances. No specific machine requirements are necessary and the authors use most major vendors' products with good effect. Color Doppler imaging is mandatory and pulsed wave Doppler can be extremely useful.

Transducer sterilization

There probably are three accepted strategies for the sterilization of transducers, and factors influencing

Department of Abdominal Imaging, Beth Israel Deaconess Medical Center, 1 Deaconess Road, Boston, MA 02215, USA
* Corresponding author.
E-mail address: dbrennan@bidmc.harvard.edu (D.D. Brennan).

doi:10.1016/j.cult.2006.05.005

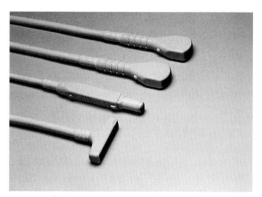

Fig. 1. IOUS is performed best with an end-fire transducer, which complements the anatomy of the gland. A wide variety of transducers is available, incorporating side-fire and end-fire designs and which have several different footprints. In most clinical situations, a standard end-fire transducer with variable frequencies can be used to good effect but occasionally specialized transducers can be used.

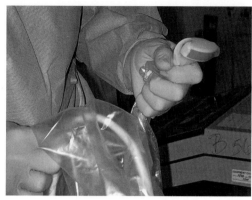

Fig. 2. A tightly fitting sheath ensures good acoustic coupling and lessens the chance of the sheath tearing during the procedure. Custom designed sheaths work best. It is important to avoid the introduction of potential imaging artifacts by ensuring even covering of the transducer surface by coupling gel.

choices include local preferences, turnover, and clinical demand on the transducers and the preference of surgical colleagues. The authors previously have used, and had excellent success using, gas sterilization with ethylene oxide for many intraoperative probes. Many manufacturers, however, are reluctant to allow gas sterilization, fearing that the transducers will be damaged by the high temperatures of aeration that are required by ethylene oxide gas sterilization, although the authors have not experienced any problems.

Another strategy involves the use of glutaraldehyde for probe sterilization, but some institutions do not consider this sufficiently sterile for open intraoperative use, and reports exist of adverse patient and staff contrast reactions to the glutaraldehyde, which can occur particularly if the probes are not rinsed sufficiently before patient exposure. At the authors' institution, direct patient contact with glutaraldehyde-soaked equipment is not allowed and, therefore, sterile probe covers are used. The application of probe covers invariably lengthens the time of the procedure by 1 or 2 minutes, and there is some risk of compromise of sterile technique if a probe cover tears, which occurs occasionally. It is preferable to use specifically designed transducer sheaths that fit snugly over the transducer head (Fig. 2), as loose fitting covers may cause imaging artifacts resulting from trapped gas or folds in the sheath. Standard endoscopic sheaths can be used to cover the entire transducer cord (Fig. 3).

The authors' preferred method of sterilization is the Sterrad system, which is gas-plasma technology using low temperature sterilization, thereby avoiding some of the problems with the high-temperature ethylene oxide systems. Sterilization is adequate to allow direct patient contact with the probes, avoiding the necessity for probe covers. There are no hazardous emissions and, hence, sterilization time is shorter, because prolonged aeration and ventilation are not required.

Who should perform intraoperative ultrasound?

In the authors' opinion, IOUS is performed best by scrubbed radiologists personally. Radiologists have scanning skills that are superior to surgeons' and also are likely to be more familiar with the ultrasound appearances of the relevant radiologic anatomy and pathology. Ultrasound is a dynamic modality, involving close hand-eye coordination learned through experience and repeated scanning, which is difficult for busy surgeons to acquire.

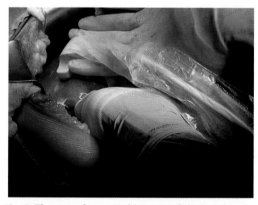

Fig. 3. The transducer cord is covered during the procedure, which enables the transducer to be introduced safely into the operative field. Sterile technique must be observed by radiologists throughout their visits to the operating suite.

Although IOUS, by its nature, removes many of the barriers to good image acquisition, such as noise from overlying structures, many lesions are subtle and more likely to be missed if imaging is performed by a surgeon and interpreted either at the bedside or by remote telemetry by a radiologist. Real-time interpretation is essential, whichever method is chosen by individual institutions. If radiologists perform the scanning personally, they are able to dynamically interact with and assess the local imaging environment and, thus, lessen the chance of inappropriate imaging parameters being chosen. Radiologists can be certain that the entire gland and surrounding area are imaged and that appropriate transducer, gain, and focal zone settings are obtained.

In an era of unparalleled growth in imaging volume, the time burden of IOUS is believed by many radiologists and practices to be onerous, but adherence to a few basic principals and incorporation of a few little tricks can minimize the time necessary to perform and interpret these studies. The most important factor in reducing time burden is to have advance notice that an IOUS case is going to happen. This enables the remainder of the schedule to be arranged accordingly. At the authors' institution, a technologist takes the scanner with the protective sheaths and appropriate transducers at the time of commencement of the surgical procedure. Radiologists performing the procedure arrive at work in surgical scrubs, thus lessening time required for changing. There is a standard arrangement with the surgeons that they call no more than 15 minutes before the time that it is anticipated the radiologists are needed and there is a reciprocal guarantee that the radiologists arrive no later than 15 minutes after that call. Although this arrangement works well in academic departments where staff are available to cross-cover and supervise residents and fellows, this model might work less well in busy practice environments. Nevertheless, by devising a model that works well for individual institutions, an IOUS service can be offered to surgeons, ensuring maximal patient care while building important relationships with surgical colleagues. Scrubbing and placing the protective sheaths take approximately 10 minutes and actual scanning usually takes no more than 5 to 10 minutes. In this way, with careful planning, IOUS can be performed in approximately 30 minutes in total.

Intraoperative scanning technique

The entire pancreatic gland is scanned in a systematic manner after adequate exposure by a surgeon. Intraoperative scanning of the pancreas can be performed entirely with the gland in situ or after surgical kocherization is performed. The body and tail are exposed by mobilizing omentum off the transverse colon and dividing adhesions between the stomach and pancreas. The transducer is held between two fingers (Fig. 4). The transducer is applied lightly to the surface of the gland using natural moisture as a coupling agent and the entire gland then is examined in transverse and sagittal planes, using multiple overlapping sweeps to ensure coverage of the entire gland. The gland should not be supported manually, as natural landmarks, such as veins and arteries, are distorted. In addition, it is important not to compress the gland with the transducer, as superficial lesions may be distorted. If a superficial lesion is suspected, the field can be flooded with sterile saline or degassed water, which can serve as a stand-off (Fig. 5) [2]. It is important to be satisfied that the entire gland, including the distal tail and uncinate process, is scanned. Lesions identified should be confirmed in two planes, and their relationship to surrounding vessels and biliary ducts, bowel, and pancreatic duct ascertained. If kocherization has not occurred, the left lobe of the liver (Fig. 6) sometimes can be used as an acoustic window, as can compressed bowel, but the images rendered are less satisfactory than when the transducer is placed directly on the gland. A lower frequency transducer frequently also is necessary. If a pancreatic neoplasm is found, the liver should be evaluated with IOUS also to rule out metastatic disease.

Relevant surgical anatomy

The anatomy of the pancreas and its anatomic relationships should already be familiar to radiologists. The pancreas is derived anatomically from a dorsal and ventral anlage that fuse after extensive in utero

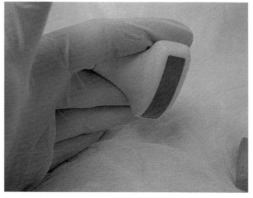

Fig. 4. The transducer is held lightly between two fingers in an operator's dominant hand and a series of overlapping transaxial and sagittal images are acquired ensuring that the entire are of interest is covered.

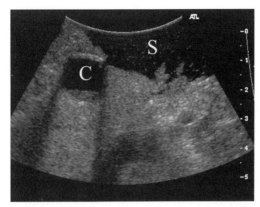

Fig. 5. If a superficial lesion is suspected, the imaging field can be flooded with sterile degassed saline, which has favorable properties as a coupling agent and for acoustic transmission, enabling the near field to be evaluated accurately. The near field has been flooded by saline (S). The cystic lesion (C) proved to represent a benign mucinous neoplasm at surgery.

rotation. The pancreas usually is slightly hyperechoic to surrounding liver parenchyma. With age and in cases of fatty infiltration, the gland can become quite hyperechoic and, although this usually is diffuse, more regional or focal fatty infiltration,

particularly in the regions of the neck or the dorsal anlage [3], can occur. As the echogenicity of the pancreas gland can vary widely, the echogenicity of pancreatic tumors relative to the gland also can vary significantly and isoechoic tumors in particular can be problematic. The gland is lobulated in up to 20% of patients and invaginations of retroperitoneal fat occasionally can be misinterpreted as focal surface lesions [4]. An echogenic, fat-replaced pancreas can be difficult to distinguish from the background retroperitoneal fat and, in these cases, reference to surrounding vessels can be used to approximate the pancreatic boundaries.

The pancreas lies in the anterior pararenal space. There are multiple arteries in close relationship to the gland. The splenic artery runs laterally along the posterior surface of the body and tail of the pancreas, although this artery has a variable course and can run through the pancreatic parenchyma as a normal variant in some patients. The gastroduodenal artery runs in a craniocaudad direction along the superolateral portion of the head. The superior mesenteric artery (SMA) runs inferior to the neck. Multiple veins are seen in close relationship to the pancreas. The superior mesenteric vein (SMV) runs anterolateral to the SMA, maintaining a course between the uncinate process behind and the pancreatic neck in front. The splenic vein courses from left to right along the dorsal margin of the pancreas and has a much more constant course than the artery (Figs. 7 and 8). The multiple arterial and venous arcades that surround the pancreatic head usually are

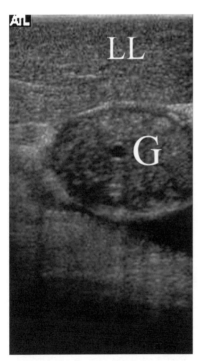

Fig. 6. Intraoperative image of autoimmune pancreatitis. The left lobe of the liver (LL) has been used as an acoustic window to evaluate the enlarged hypoechoic gland (G). Decompressed stomach, duodenum, and the left lobe of the liver are used as acoustic windows during IOUS.

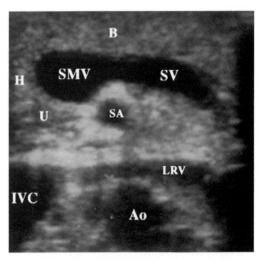

Fig. 7. Normal intraoperative anatomy of the pancreas. Note that the parenchyma in this case is relatively hyperechoic. Transaxial image reveals the body (B), head (H), and uncinate process (U) of the pancreas and their relationship to the splenic vein (SV), SMV, left renal vein (LRV), aorta (Ao), and inferior vena cava (IVC).

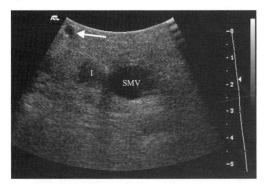

Fig. 8. In another patient who had a small insulinoma (I), the relationship of the pancreatic neck to the gastroduodenal artery (*arrow*) is appreciated clearly. Note the patient's SMV.

not resolved at IOUS imaging. When evaluating the vessels, attention to replaced or accessory hepatic arteries off the SMA should be made, as these vessels can be ligated accidentally at the time of cholecystectomy performed as part of the Whipple procedure. In addition to these, assessment for significant arterial stenoses of the SMA or, more importantly, celiac axis should be made, as an occluded celiac axis can preclude a successful Whipple procedure [5]. Furthermore, significant ectasia or calcifications of the splenic artery should be identified, as a healthy pancreaticojejunal anastomosis depends on this artery and its main dorsal pancreatic branch. The pancreatic duct measures less than 3 mm and has a variable course through the pancreas. When less than 1 mm, the duct appears as an echogenic line. Duct stenoses and dilatations are seen in chronic pancreatitis, but studies from the endoscopic retrograde cholangiopancreatography (ERCP) literature suggest a long differential [6]. Strictures more than 1 cm are more suggestive of malignancy.

Artifacts, variants, and other potential pitfalls

Recognition of artifacts—technical and from anatomic and pathologic structures—is essential to performing and interpreting IOUS studies correctly. In addition to artifacts already familiar to radiologists who perform transabdominal ultrasound of the pancreas, specific IOUS pitfalls exist. Common mistakes include misinterpreting vascular calcifications as parenchymal classifications and, thus, erroneously assigning a diagnosis of chronic pancreatitis. As discussed previously, it is important to recognize accessory arteries from the SMA. Similarly, pseudoaneurysms and pseudocysts can be confused if Doppler color flow imaging is not used (Fig. 9A,B), and, as both occur commonly in the context of acute pancreatitis, color Doppler evaluation of all such lesions is recommended before aspiration (Fig. 10A,B). Duodenal lesions, diverticulae, and thickening can be misidentified as coming from the pancreas and distal pancreatic lesions occasionally can be misassigned to the left adrenal gland as the gland may lie behind the splenic vein in this location. As discussed previously, fatty infiltration or lobulation can be misinterpreted as a true lesion. Other peripancreatic lesions that potentially could be misinterpreted as intrapancreatic include peripancreatic lymph nodes, focal pancreatitis, and aberrant vessels, although Doppler and color flow imaging should allow vessels to be characterized accurately. Specific problems that can occur with IOUS include artifacts from a poorly fitting sheath

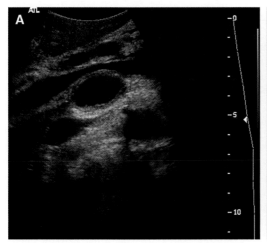
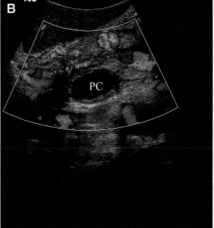

Fig. 9. IOUS performed in a patient who had acute and chronic pancreatitis. Multiple hypoechoic structures are identified on gray scale imaging (*A*). After the application of color flow, the pancreatic pseudocyst (PC) can be differentiated from the background vasculature (*B*).

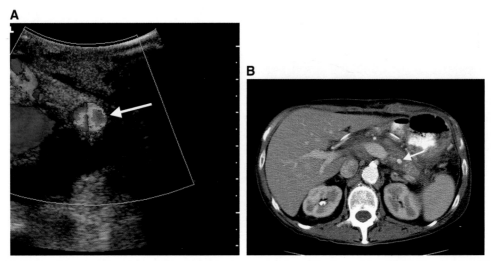

A

B

Fig. 10. IOUS with color flow in a patient who had acute pancreatitis. To-and-fro blood flow is identified in a rounded lesion (*arrow*) (*A*) that proved to represent a small splenic artery pseudoaneurysm at MDCT (*arrow*) (*B*).

or poor coupling on an irregular surface. Radiologists need to be conscious that lesions in the near field are easy to overlook in IOUS. Finally, remember that pancreatic carcinoma and focal pancreatitis can, and frequently do, coexist [7].

Clinical applications

Inflammatory disorders of the pancreas

Acute pancreatitis

Acute pancreatitis, from whatever cause, frequently is complicated by pseudocyst and abscess formation. Surgical treatment of these lesions frequently is necessary and can involve cystgastrostomy or cystenterostomy [8] formation and débridement and necrosectomy. Pseudocysts frequently are multiple and do not always communicate with each other or with the pancreatic duct; thus, IOUS can have a valuable role in identifying multiple small pseudocysts and guiding aspiration of them [9]. This is true especially of pseudocysts in unusual locations, such as around the duodenum, porta hepatis, and spleen (Fig. 11) [10,11]. Furthermore, vital vascular structures can be avoided and pseudoaneurysms identified correctly. In cases of traumatic pancreatitis or transection, the pancreatic ductal anatomy can be identified [12]. Cysts and pseudocysts also can be recognized easily [13] and characterized as either simple or complex by IOUS, which may alter treatment (Fig. 12) [14]. Gallstones and common duct stones and gravel [15] can be identified, thus directing the need for intraoperative common bile duct exploration or postoperative therapeutic ERCP. Finally, the pancreas can be evaluated for other causes, such as small tumors and rare ductal

anomalies, for instance, duplication [16] and pancreatic divisum.

Chronic pancreatitis

One of the major surgical treatments of chronic pancreatitis is the lateral pancreaticojejunostomy, or Puestow procedure, in which the pancreatic duct is filleted open and a side-to-side anastomosis is performed with a loop of jejunum. The larger the duct, the easier the procedure is for surgeons to perform. IOUS can be used in many ways to assist surgeons as part of this procedure. In the simplest way,

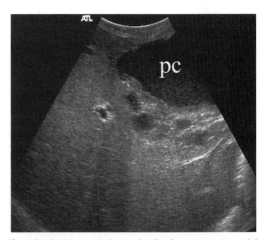

Fig. 11. IOUS in a patient who had acute pancreatitis revealed a large pseudocyst (PC), which dissected into the liver. IOUS was used to guide safe surgical decompression and to delineate the relevant hepatic and portal vasculature. Internal debris can be detected easily with the fine spatial and contrast resolution inherent to the intraoperative technique.

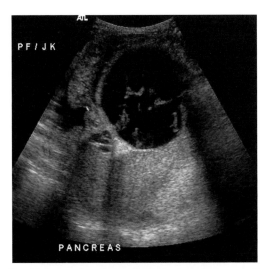

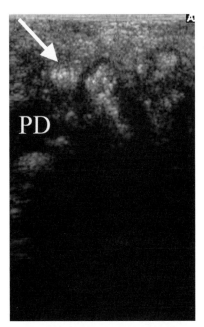

Fig. 12. In another patient who had acute pancreatitis, a large complex pseudocyst is identified with significant internal debris and septations. The determination of the complexity of these lesions is important in guiding therapy, as more complex pseudocysts are less likely to respond to simple aspiration. The relationship of these pseudocysts to the pancreatic duct should be established in each case, where possible.

Fig. 13. In a patient who had chronic pancreatitis, IOUS elegantly delineates an intraductal calculus (*arrow*). If bypass is being performed, this calculus needs to be removed surgically or else the bypass needs to be performed proximal to this obstructing calculus. PD, pancreatic duct.

the course of the pancreatic duct, which is variable at the best of times and unpredictable in chronic pancreatitis, is assessed by a radiologist and a suitable point, where the duct superficially, is marked. If there are intraductal calculi present, they can be removed or a point proximal to an obstructing calculus can be used for drainage (Fig. 13). A surgeon cuts down at this point to the duct [17]. Alternatively, and preferably, the duct can be cannulated with a needle by a radiologist (or surgeon) under direct sonographic visualization (Figs. 14 and 15). This enables the surgeon to cut down along the course of the needle to the duct. Aspiration can be performed to confirm that the needle is intaductal. In a further extension of this technique, some groups use this needle to cannulate the duct with a wire [18,19] (which subsequently is threaded retrogradely into the proximal duct), providing surgeons with more stability. In the authors' experience, cannulation with a 27-G needle works well and is the preferred method. IOUS localization of the pancreatic duct saves considerable operating room time, because the rock-hard fibrotic pancreas prevents accurate localization by palpation.

In some patients who have chronic pancreatitis, diffuse ductal sclerosis and narrowing occur. Many of these cases reflect autoimmune pancreatitis and can be steroid responsive [20]. In lymphoplasmacytic sclerosing pancreatitis, the entire gland shows an abnormal heterogenous echotexture at IOUS and, if recognized, this can be confirmed by

intraoperative biopsy (Fig. 16). In patients who have nonautoimmune chronic pancreatitis, where no discrete point of obstruction is identified, and in patients who have diffuse parenchymal calcification and obliteration, surgeons may elect to

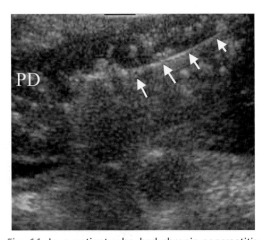

Fig. 14. In a patient who had chronic pancreatitis, IOUS has been used to guide a small needle (*arrows*) into the pancreatic duct (PD). A surgeon then can cut down onto this needle and ensure that the pancreatic duct is exposed adequately before performing a Puestow procedure (pancreaticojejunostomy). In patients who have chronic pancreatitis, this simple maneuver saves significant time.

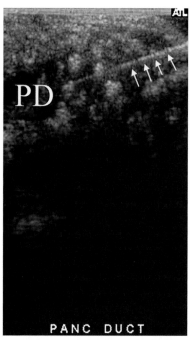

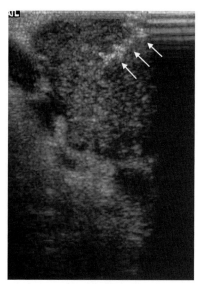

Fig. 16. Intraoperative laparascopic ultrasound–guided biopsy of an abnormal enlarged pancreas that proved to represent lymphoplasmocytic autoimmune pancreatitis. The needle can be identified extending into the heterogeneously enlarged gland (*arrows*).

Fig. 15. In another patient who had chronic pancreatitis, a needle (*arrows*) has been advanced into a pancreatic duct (PD) that is dilated and filled with echogenic debris and multiple small calculi. Calculi in chronic pancreatitis often do not calcify. This simple maneuver saves significant time in patients who have chronic pancreatitis, as the duct frequently is difficult to identify in this patient population because of scarring and inflammation.

perform a subtotal pancreatectomy rather than a Puestow procedure. This information can be obtained easily at the time of IOUS (Fig. 17) [21].

Tumor localization and staging

Pancreatic adenocarcinoma

Pancreatic adenocarcinoma is the fourth leading cause of cancer deaths in men and women in the United States. Of the gastrointestinal malignancies, it is the second leading cause of death. The American Cancer Society estimates that in 2005, 32,000 Americans will be diagnosed with adenocarcinoma of the pancreas and approximately 31,000 will die of the disease [22]. Approximately 20% to 40% of patients who have pancreatic cancer seem to have the cancer contained entirely within the pancreas at the time of the diagnosis. Surgical removal of the tumor is recommended in this group of patients and this provides the best option for long-term survival.

Vascular invasion usually precludes a successful pancreatic resection or at the least mandates the use of bypass grafts, significantly complicating an already difficult procedure. Preoperative staging

can be performed using several competing and complementary modalities, including CT, MR imaging, and endoscopic ultrasound [23]. IOUS also has a role in the management of pancreatic adenocarcinoma. It is extremely useful for the identification of nonpalpable tumors, which, although rare, do occur, particularly in the context of pancreatitis, and also for defining the relationship of tumors to adjacent vital structures [24,25]. Earlier studies suggest that IOUS influences or alters surgical management

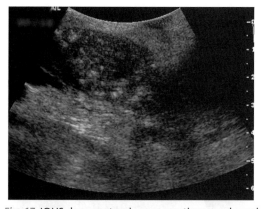

Fig. 17. IOUS shows extensive pancreatic parenchymal calcification in a patient who had chronic pancreatitis. No significant pancreatic ductal dilatation is appreciated, so a lateral pancreaticojejunostomy (Puestow procedure) technically becomes extremely difficult.

in up to one third [26] to one half [24] of cases, but as alternative imaging modalities have improved, their sensitivities and specificities for the assessment of disease resectability also have improved and IOUS is not likely to have such a significant effect currently. At the authors' institution, laparoscopy is performed before open surgery and laparascopic ultrasound of the pancreas, peripancreatic area, and liver is performed at this time. This combined approach of laparoscopic visualization of the peritoneum and mesentery and liver surface, coupled with laparoscopic ultrasound assessment of the SMA, SMV, and hepatic vessels and preoperative staging multidetector CT (MDCT), minimizes the number of patients subjected to open surgery who ultimately prove unresectable [23], although IOUS still can depict the relationship of tumors to vessels elegantly (Fig. 18). Adenocarcinomas usually are hypoechoic and lesions as small as 3 mm can be detected by IOUS (Fig. 19). Complications of adenocarcinoma, such as ductal obstruction, nodes, and hepatic metastases, also can be detected readily at IOUS (Fig. 20) [24,26].

Cystic neoplasms of the pancreas

Cystic neoplasms can be identified easily at IOUS and impressive spatial resolution allows their internal architecture to be characterized exquisitely [27]. Surface or internal calcifications, mural papillary excrescences, pseudocapsules, and internal septations, all features of mucinous cystadenomas or cystadenocarcinomas, are identified readily (Fig. 21A,B). The tumor margins and relationships to surrounding vessels are defined easily and IOUS also can be used to guide percutaneous needle aspiration for assessment of mucin content and

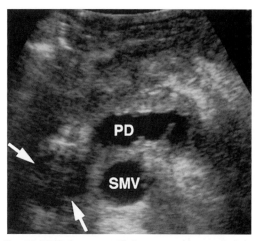

Fig. 19. IOUS shows a well-demarcated hypoechoic lesion in head of the pancreas (*arrows*). Note the pancreatic duct (PD) dilatation.

tumor markers [9]. Benign serous tumors are lobulated tumors with thick fibrous capsules but should not contain septae or mural irregularities. Internally, multiple small (2-mm) simple cysts are present, which usually appear echogenic on transcutaneous ultrasound because of many internal reflections from cyst walls (Fig. 22). The presence of a central stellate fibrous scar with calcifications,

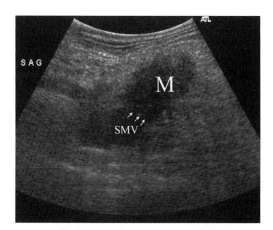

Fig. 18. Adenocarcinoma invading the SMV. A focal hypoechoic lesion (M) surrounds almost 50% of the lateral wall of the SMV (*arrows*). This lesion was unresectable at the time of surgery.

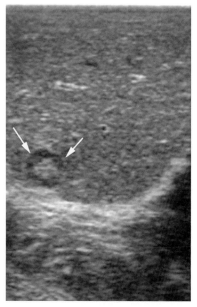

Fig. 20. IOUS of the liver performed at the time of pancreatic adenocarcinoma resection shows a small parenchymal lesion (*arrows*) that proved to represent a metastasis at intraoperative biopsy. A planned Whipple procedure was abandoned.

A   B

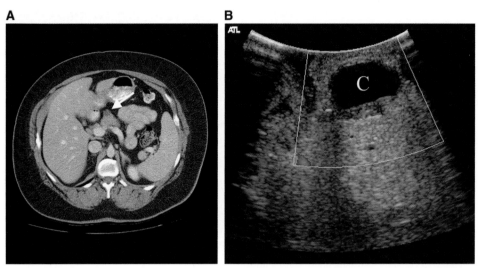

Fig. 21. (*A, B*) Preoperative CT examination reveals an exophytic hypodense lesion (*arrow*). At IOUS, this was shown to be a thick-walled cystic lesion with some dependent layering (C). Preoperative sampling under endoscopic ultrasound had revealed a carcinoembryonic antigen level of 22,000. Final histology after resection was of a benign mucinous cystadenoma.

a typical imaging feature, can be appreciated by IOUS.

Intraductal pancreatic mucinous tumors

Intraductal pancreatic mucinous tumors (IPMTs) are other tumors that lend themselves well to IOUS assessment [28]. These neoplasms can be divided into either main branch type or side branch type [29]. The former usually requires a total pancreatectomy, but side branch tumors can be treated by watchful waiting [30] or local excision, often with curative intent, as these frequently are low-grade neoplasms [31,32]. IOUS can be used to define the extent of the disease intraoperatively (Fig. 23A,B) and, thus, guide the extent of surgical resection required [28]. Small intraductal

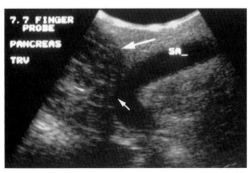

Fig. 22. In a patient who had a microcystic (serous) adenocarcinoma (*arrows*), IOUS elegantly delineates the multiple small echogenic layers that reflect the walls of the multiple small constituent cysts.

hyperechoic side branch neoplasms are visualized well at IOUS. Meticulous attention to detail can enable surgeons to obtain clear margins confidently while minimizing morbidity and preserving adequate endocrine and exocrine pancreatic function.

Tumors arising from islet cells

IOUS has an invaluable role to play in the localization of islet cell tumors. These tumors are derived from the islets of Langherhans and those that are hormonally active frequently present with characteristic clinical syndromes at a time when the tumor is very small. Alpha cells produce glucagon, and glucagonomas frequently are single, are malignant, and present with refractory hyperglycemia with or without a pathognomic rash (necrolytic migratory erythema). Insulinomas are the most common and are produced by beta cells from the islets of Langherhans. They present with spontaneous hypoglycemia. Most IOUS experience is with this tumor. As patients clinically present early, the tumor tends to be small. Up to 20% are nonpalpable and, in these cases, IOUS can be invaluable in detecting the tumor [2,33,34]. Insulinomas tend to be benign, so surgical treatment is definitive. After localization, IOUS can be used to define the relationship of the tumor to the pancreatic duct, as this relationship determines surgical approach. If the tumor is superficial and away from the gland, a simple enucleation can be performed, but if it is related closely to the gland, a pancreatic gland excision needs to be undertaken, with increased morbidity [35]. By evaluating the relationship of the tumor to the duct,

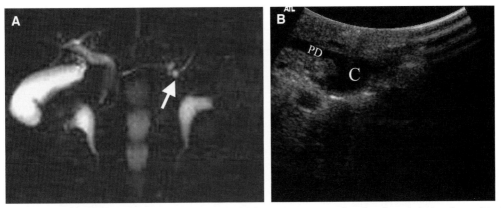

Fig. 23. Side branch IPMT. (*A*) A single, coronal thick slab MR image reveals a focal cystic lesion (*arrow*) in the midbody of the pancreas, which seems continuous with the main pancreatic duct. (*B*) IOUS in the same patient confirms the presence of the cystic lesion (C) and its direct continuity with the main pancreatic duct (PD). IOUS was used to define the margins of the tumor for resection.

complications, such as postoperative fistulas and collections, can be lessened. Intraoperative biopsy also can be performed under IOUS, but this rarely is necessary. Most insulinomas tend to be hypoechoic to the background parenchyma, but up to 10% may be hyperechoic or isoechoic (Fig. 24) [36]. Isoechoic lesions tend to occur in younger patients and represent a diagnostic challenge. Distortion of local anatomy or recognition of halos or pseudocapsules, refractive shadows, or fine internal septations can enable their visualization. When evaluating patients who have insulinoma, it is important to evaluate the entire gland, even after the index lesion is identified, because in patients who have multiple endocrine neoplasia (MEN)-1, the tumors may be multiple. These multiple tumors are very small, and these patients usually can be

identified by clinical history and by the demonstration of tumors elsewhere. The surgical approach often is to perform a distal pancreatectomy combined with enucleation of any proximal tumors. As with any pancreatic tumor, evaluation of the peripancreatic area for lymphadenopathy, the liver for metastases, and pancreatic vessels for signs of unresectability is mandatory, although insulinomas tend for the most part to be benign.

Gastrinomas frequently are extrapancreatic (20%–40%), malignant (60%–90%), and large and multiple (20%–40%). The "gastrinoma triangle" is the site where most extrapancreatic gastrinomas lie and is bounded by the second and third parts of the duodenum, the common duct, and the head of the pancreas. In patients who have symptoms of this disease, IOUS evaluation of the

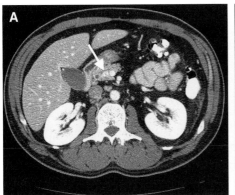
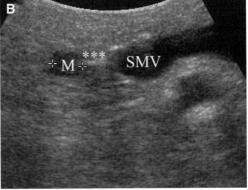

Fig. 24. (*A*) CT performed in a patient who had spontaneous hypoglycemia shows a small hypervascular lesion that proved on resection to represent an insulinoma (*arrow*). (*B*) IOUS showed the nonpalpable lesion (M) between measuring callipers and its relationship to the SMV. The artifact from air between the lesion and the SMV (*asterisks*) was from surgical dissection along the proposed plane of cleavage. The lesion was treated successfully by a partial pancreatectomy.

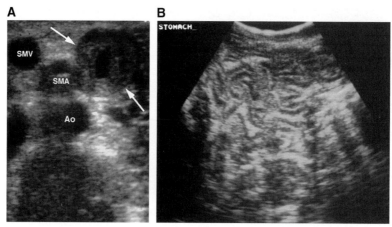

Fig. 25. (*A*) IOUS in a patient who had a gastrinoma shows a hypoechoic lymph node metastasis (*arrows*). Although sensitivities are lower than with intrapancreatic lesions, IOUS still is a useful adjunct to surgical palpations for identifying intra- and extrapancreatic islet cell tumors. (*B*) In another patient who had Zollinger-Ellison syndrome secondary to a malignant gastrinoma, extensive thickening of the stomach wall is identified at the time of IOUS secondary to excessive acid production inherent to this condition. Ao, aorta.

wall of the duodenum and this region is mandatory (Fig. 25) [37]. Gastrinomas frequently are associated with MEN-1 and, in this context, also frequently are multiple. IOUS is more successful in locating intrapancreatic tumors—where success rates are only slightly lower than for insulinomas—than extrapancreatic tumors—where the success rate falls significantly [38–40].

Werner-Morrison syndrome (watery diarrhea, hypokalemia, acidosis) usually is the clinical presentation of a VIPoma. IOUS experience with this tumor and with somatostatinomas is limited. As these lesions and the so-called "nonfunctioning" islet cell tumors often present as large masses, the role of IOUS often is limited. These tumors, however, even when metastatic, frequently are more plastic than adenocarcinomas and do not demonstrate the same degree of vascular or neural invasion. They frequently are well marginated and tend to be locally resectable.

Summary

IOUS is placed ideally to facilitate diagnosing and guide treatment of several important and common pancreatic conditions, inflammatory and neoplastic. Its high contrast and spatial resolution, coupled with its ability to guide intraoperatively, make it indispensable to pancreatic surgeons. It has a significant influence on patient care and surgical decision-making. In the authors' opinion, it is a technique performed best by scrubbed radiologists and can be implemented in daily practice without having an undue impact on work flow.

References

[1] Lane RJ, Glazer G. Intra-operative B-mode ultrasound scanning of the extra-hepatic biliary system and pancreas. Lancet 1980;2:334.

[2] Grant CS, van Heerden J, Charboneau JW, et al. Insulinoma. The value of intraoperative ultrasonography. Arch Surg 1988;123:843.

[3] Atri M, Nazarnia S, Mehio A, et al. Hypoechogenic embryologic ventral aspect of the head and uncinate process of the pancreas: in vitro correlation of US with histopathologic findings. Radiology 1994;190:441.

[4] Ross BA, Jeffrey RB Jr, Mindelzun RE. Normal variations in the lateral contour of the head and neck of the pancreas mimicking neoplasm: evaluation with dual-phase helical CT. AJR Am J Roentgenol 1996;166:799.

[5] Strasberg SM, Drebin JA, Mokadam NA, et al. Prospective trial of a blood supply-based technique of pancreaticojejunostomy: effect on anastomotic failure in the Whipple procedure. J Am Coll Surg 2002;194:746.

[6] Rohrmann CA, Silvis SE, Vennes JA. The significance of pancreatic ductal obstruction in differential diagnosis of the abnormal endoscopic retrograde pancreatogram. Radiology 1976;121:311.

[7] Imamura M, Asahi S, Yamauchi H, et al. Minute pancreatic carcinoma with initial symptom of acute pancreatitis. J Hepatobiliary Pancreat Surg 2002;9:632.

[8] Altimari A, Aranha GV, Greenlee HB, et al. Results of cystoduodenostomy for treatment of pancreatic pseudocysts. Am Surg 1986;52:438.

[9] Machi J, Sigel B, Kurohiji T, et al. Operative ultrasound guidance for various surgical procedures. Ultrasound Med Biol 1990;16:37.

[10] Gooding GA, Linkowski GD, Deveney C, et al. Intraoperative sonography of perisplenic pseudocysts. AJR Am J Roentgenol 1985;145:1013.

[11] Rindsberg S, Radecki PD, Friedman AC, et al. Intraoperative ultrasonic localization of a small pancreatic pseudocyst. Gastrointest Radiol 1986;11:339.

[12] Hikida S, Sakamoto T, Higaki K, et al. Intraoperative ultrasonography is useful for diagnosing pancreatic duct injury and adjacent tissue damage in a patient with penetrating pancreas trauma. J Hepatobiliary Pancreat Surg 2004;11:272.

[13] Kurohiji T, Sigel B, Machi J, et al. Detection of preoperatively unrecognized multiple pancreatic pseudocysts by intraoperative ultrasonography. Report of two cases. Am Surg 1991;57:668.

[14] Ros PR, Hamrick-Turner JE, Chiechi MV, et al. Cystic masses of the pancreas. Radiographics 1992;12:673.

[15] Machi J, Sigel B, Zaren HA, et al. Operative ultrasonography during hepatobiliary and pancreatic surgery. World J Surg 1993;17:640.

[16] Ohkubo T, Imamura H, Sugawara Y, et al. Successful pancreatic duct-to-jejunum anastomosis in a patient with a double pancreatic duct: usefulness of intraoperative ultrasonography (IOUS) and IOUS-guided pancreatography. Hepatogastroenterology 2002;49:1724.

[17] Machi J, Sigel B, Kodama I, et al. Ultrasound-guided pancreatotomy for opening the pancreatic duct. Surg Gynecol Obstet 1991;173:59.

[18] Mayo-Smith WW, Iannitti DA, Dupuy DE. Intraoperative sonographically guided wire cannulation of the pancreatic duct for patients undergoing a Puestow procedure. AJR Am J Roentgenol 2000;175:1639.

[19] Noike T, Miyagawa S, Shimada R, et al. Securing a small-caliber pancreatic duct for longitudinal pancreatojejunostomy. Hepatogastroenterology 2002;49:1139.

[20] Wakabayashi T, Kawaura Y, Satomura Y, et al. Long-term prognosis of duct-narrowing chronic pancreatitis: strategy for steroid treatment. Pancreas 2005;30:31.

[21] Printz H, Klotter HJ, Nies C, et al. Intraoperative ultrasonography in surgery for chronic pancreatitis. Int J Pancreatol 1992;12:233.

[22] http://www.cancer.org, ACS. 2005. Accessed April 6, 2006.

[23] Long EE, Van Dam J, Weinstein S, et al. Computed tomography, endoscopic, laparoscopic, and intraoperative sonography for assessing resectability of pancreatic cancer. Surg Oncol 2005;14:105.

[24] Serio G, Fugazzola C, Iacono C, et al. Intraoperative ultrasonography in pancreatic cancer. Int J Pancreatol 1992;11:31.

[25] Alberti A, Dattola P, Littori F, et al. [Intraoperative ultrasonography in the staging of pancreatic head neoplasms]. Chir Ital 2002;54:59.

[26] Flati G, Flati D, Porowska B, et al. Is intraoperative ultrasonography useful in pancreatic cancer surgery? G Chir 1994;15:313.

[27] Kubota K, Noie T, Sano K, et al. Impact of intraoperative ultrasonography on surgery for cystic lesions of the pancreas. World J Surg 1997;21:72.

[28] Kaneko T, Nakao A, Inoue S, et al. Intraoperative ultrasonography by high-resolution annular array transducer for intraductal papillary mucinous tumors of the pancreas. Surgery 2001; 129:55.

[29] Procacci C, Graziani R, Bicego E, et al. Intraductal mucin-producing tumors of the pancreas: imaging findings. Radiology 1996;198:249.

[30] Irie H, Yoshimitsu K, Aibe H, et al. Natural history of pancreatic intraductal papillary mucinous tumor of branch duct type: follow-up study by magnetic resonance cholangiopancreatography. J Comput Assist Tomogr 2004;28:117.

[31] Paye F, Sauvanet A, Terris B, et al. Intraductal papillary mucinous tumors of the pancreas: pancreatic resections guided by preoperative morphological assessment and intraoperative frozen section examination. Surgery 2000;127:536.

[32] Terris B, Ponsot P, Paye F, et al. Intraductal papillary mucinous tumors of the pancreas confined to secondary ducts show less aggressive pathologic features as compared with those involving the main pancreatic duct. Am J Surg Pathol 2000;24:1372.

[33] Hiramoto JS, Feldstein VA, LaBerge JM, et al. Intraoperative ultrasound and preoperative localization detects all occult insulinomas. Arch Surg 2001;136:1020 [discussion: 1025–6].

[34] Kuzin NM, Egorov AV, Kondrashin SA, et al. Preoperative and intraoperative topographic diagnosis of insulinomas. World J Surg 1998;22:593.

[35] Park BJ, Alexander HR, Libutti SK, et al. Operative management of islet-cell tumors arising in the head of the pancreas. Surgery 1998; 124:1056.

[36] Gorman B, Charboneau JW, James EM, et al. Benign pancreatic insulinoma: preoperative and intraoperative sonographic localization. AJR Am J Roentgenol 1986;147:929.

[37] Kisker O, Bastian D, Bartsch D, et al. Localization, malignant potential, and surgical management of gastrinomas. World J Surg 1998;22:651.

[38] Sugg SL, Norton JA, Fraker DL, et al. A prospective study of intraoperative methods to diagnose and resect duodenal gastrinomas. Ann Surg 1993;218:138.

[39] Norton JA. Intraoperative methods to stage and localize pancreatic and duodenal tumors. Ann Oncol 1999;10(Suppl 4):182.

[40] Norton JA, Cromack DT, Shawker TH, et al. Intraoperative ultrasonographic localization of islet cell tumors. A prospective comparison to palpation. Ann Surg 1988;207:160.

ULTRASOUND
CLINICS

Ultrasound Clin 1 (2006) 547–557

Intraoperative Laparoscopic Ultrasound

Suvranu Ganguli, MD[a,b,]*, Jonathan B. Kruskal, MD, PhD[a,b],
Darren D. Brennan, MD[a,b], Robert A. Kane, MD, FACR[a,b]

- ▪ Laparoscopic probe design
- ▪ Transducer sterilization
- ▪ Intraoperative scanning techniques
- ▪ Operating room ergonomics
- ▪ Clinical applications of laparoscopic ultrasound

  Laparoscopic ultrasound of the liver

Laparoscopic ultrasound of the gallbladder and bile ducts
Laparoscopic ultrasound of the pancreas
Other applications
- ▪ Biopsy and percutaneous ablation guidance
- ▪ Summary
- ▪ References

As minimally invasive surgery and laparoscopic alternatives to open surgical procedures continue to increase, the demand for and use of intraoperative laparoscopic ultrasound (LUS) techniques also are increasing steadily. The benefit of scanning directly on the surface of intra-abdominal organs, structures, and pathology and the improved spatial and contrast resolution seen in open intraoperative ultrasound (IOUS) [1] can be transferred to laparoscopic procedures. LUS shows beneficial applications in evaluating normal structures and pathology within the liver, pancreas, biliary tract, and gallbladder [2–4]. There also are reports of LUS improving localization and laparoscopic staging of intra-abdominal tumors [5–8]. The need for specially designed equipment, especially special transducers for LUS, traditionally has been the greatest obstacle to its widespread use. With the increasing demand and use of laparoscopy and LUS, however, there continues to be improving technology and exciting new possibilities.

Laparoscopic probe design

The overriding stipulation for laparoscopic probes is that the diameter of the imaging crystal and shaft must be small enough to be inserted through a standard laparoscopic port 10 to 11 mm in diameter. Transducer technology has progressed substantially from the first reports of LUS, where investigators used A-mode transducers to visualize intra-abdominal organs and assist in the diagnosis of intra-abdominal pathology [9,10]. The limited amount of information obtained with the primitive A-mode technology resulted in limited applicability of this technique. The subsequent development of real-time B-mode ultrasound and improved miniaturization technology made the laparoscopic approach more feasible. Early probes also used a rotating radial probe [11], but the subsequent development of linear array and curved array, high-frequency probes has resulted in superior image resolution.

[a] Department of Radiology, Beth Israel Deaconess Medical Center, 330 Brookline Avenue, Boston, MA 02215, USA
[b] Harvard Medical School, Boston, MA, USA
* Corresponding author. Department of Radiology, Beth Israel Deaconess Medical Center, 330 Brookline Avenue, Boston, MA 02215.
E-mail address: sganguli@caregroup.harvard.edu (S. Ganguli).

doi:10.1016/j.cult.2006.05.006

The miniaturization of the crystal size previously has led to probes with extremely small field of views. The small field of view of laparoscopic probes compared with standard ultrasound probes remains an obstacle, but the development and improvement of linear array and curved array probes have improved this constraint significantly. Optimal image crystal lengths for intra-abdominal laparoscopic probes range from 1.5 to 4 cm. Longer crystal lengths help provide larger images that can shorten scanning time of larger organs, such as the liver. The curved array probes also provide a more familiar sector-style image, allowing for easier orientation and greater visualization of deep anatomy in any one field.

In the authors' experience, probe frequencies centered at 5 MHz permit adequate depth of penetration to image the entire liver. Probes now are designed with multifrequency options or broadband technology, which allows a range of frequencies. This allows more flexibility in penetration to suit the specific intraoperative imaging needs. Higher frequencies of 7 to 10 MHz are more suitable for imaging the gallbladder, common bile duct (CBD), and pancreas. These improvements in probe technology, coupled with the expansion in computer power, have enabled the design and development of laparoscopic probes that now have the same image quality, resolution, Doppler, and color flow imaging capacities as standard ultrasound probes.

In addition to the miniaturization required of laparoscopic probes, a radically different probe design is needed to optimize use in a laparoscopic setting. Laparoscopic probes must be mounted at the end of a long shaft, measuring 20 to 30 cm in length, to facilitate imaging organs, structure, and pathology some distance away from the entry site on the abdominal wall (Fig. 1). Early probes were mounted on the end of rigid shafts designed to be passed through standard laparoscopic ports. Recent probes are designed to be more flexible and maneuverable at the transducer tip. At minimum, flexion and extension of the imaging crystal now are available and newer systems provide rightward and leftward steering. The flexible imaging portion of the probe allows for good tissue contact necessary for acoustic coupling to be maintained in a gas-filled peritoneal cavity. Maintaining surface contact with curved or irregularly shaped organs and mastering a maneuverable laparoscopic probe require practice and experience. Without optimal probe flexibility, adequate imaging may require filling the abdominal cavity with sterile water or saline and imaging through the fluid.

Transducer sterilization

Sterile sheaths similar to those used on standard ultrasound probes for IOUS can be used during LUS. Because of the nature of laparoscopic procedures, however, with repetitive insertion and removal of

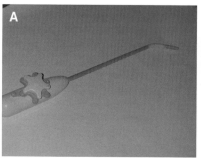
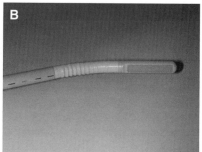
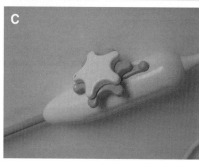

Fig. 1. Special probes (A) are required for LUS. Probes are mounted at the end of a long shaft (B) to facilitate imaging organs, structure, and pathology some distance away from the entry site on the abdominal wall. Flexion and extension of the probe is performed by turning dials (C) on the proximal shaft outside the patient.

probes through ports and using inserted tools, such as the laparoscopic instruments, for manipulation of intra-abdominal organs and structures, sheaths continually run a high risk of tearing during use. For these reasons, sterilization capability is a more optimal requirement for laparoscopic probes compared with standard ultrasound probes.

Specially designed strong sterile sheaths are used for LUS and should have a snug fit to the transducer, if used, to avoid being torn during insertion. These sheaths are long, typically approximately 1.5 m, so that the entire length of the cord can be covered. Sterile saline or gel must be used between the tip and the sheath to avoid artifact from trapped air. If sterile sheaths are used, it is still advisable to soak the probe for some time in a sterilizing solution, as the potential for tearing of the sheath and contamination of the surgical field remains.

Newer-generation laparoscopic probes are designed to be compatible with modern sterilization methods. Ideally, the entire ultrasound probe except the electronic connector is sterilized. Low-temperature hydrogen peroxide gas plasma sterilization techniques (Sterrad, Advanced Sterilization Products, Irvine, California) can complete an entire sterilization cycle in 1 to 2 hours. These sterilization techniques are safe to use with heat-sensitive equipment and can help avoid use of sterile sheaths.

Intraoperative scanning techniques

Selection of port placement is highly dependent on the target organ or area requiring LUS evaluation (Fig. 2). Often surgeons need to create port sites for the laparoscope and the laparoscopic

instruments before using LUS. Optimal placement of a port transducer site, however, usually is several centimeters away from the area to allow room to maneuver the probe freely. Frequently, the LUS probe and the laparoscope (usually in a periumbilical port) must be reversed or multiple ports must be created to reach all areas necessary with the LUS probe. If the laparoscopic procedure has the potential of being converted to an open procedure, it is optimal to include port sites within the line of a subsequent incision.

Ensuring that the ports are airtight before inserting the LUS probe is important to maintain the iatrogenic pneumoperitoneum of laparoscopy (Fig. 3). If a standard 10-mm LUS probe is inserted, make sure that the 10- to 11-mm adjustable port is set to the appropriate 10-mm size to prevent leakage of gas. After port insertion, it is important again to assess for leakage of gas around the port and address problems as they arise. The sterile transducer must be inserted carefully though the port with direct laparoscopic visualization to ensure safe delivery to the region of interest (Fig. 4). As there is no tactile sensation available to the LUS operator, direct laparoscopic visualization of the probe is imperative at all times during scanning to avoid solid organ or vessel injury. It is necessary always to be cognizant of the location of the transducer tip on the laparoscopic camera images—looking at the ultrasound image alone may cause inadvertent injury (Fig. 5).

Even though the peritoneal cavity is distended with gas, natural organ surface moisture usually is sufficient to permit adequate acoustic coupling and optimal image quality. If necessary, sterile saline can be introduced onto the organ surface to enhance acoustic coupling. As discussed previously, if an overlying sheath is used, sterile saline or gel must be used between the tip and the sheath to avoid artifact from trapped air.

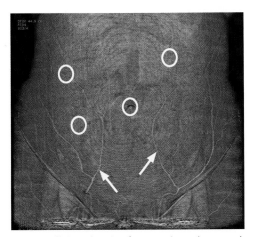

Fig. 2. Localizing the site for port insertion requires avoiding important subcutaneous vessels (*arrows*). Common insertion sites (shown as rings) are in the left and right subcostal, right lower quadrant and umbilical regions.

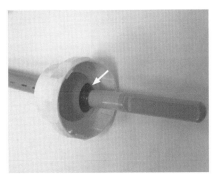

Fig. 3. The sterile transducer should create an airtight seal as it passes through the port. Note the circular valve (*arrow*), which ensures that the port is airtight.

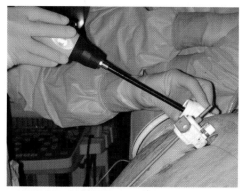

Fig. 4. The sterile transducer must be inserted carefully through the port, keeping an eye on the monitor to ensure safe delivery into a region of interest. If a sheath is used, very gentle insertion is essential to avoid tearing.

The optimal choice of imaging frequency is dependent on the target organ or organ system. The gallbladder, extrahepatic CBD, and pancreas can be imaged successfully at a 7-MHz frequency. The liver, however, is imaged optimally at a 5-MHz frequency, which penetrates to a depth of 10 to 12 cm rather than a depth of approximately 6 cm at 7 MHz. Using the lower, 5-MHz frequency does not impair the ability of visualize small lesions but does facilitate complete scanning of the liver from the anterior surface of the liver [2]. This way, using the undersurface of the liver for scanning can be avoided. The undersurface of the liver is much more irregular and less accessible, causing imaging from this side to be more challenging technically.

Compared with IOUS, LUS takes substantially more time to image the same structures because of the small crystal size and field of view. The curved array sector scanners give an impression of a large field of view, but this is true only at depths of several centimeters. The near field is limited by the transducer length, which may be as short as 1.5 to 2 cm. Therefore, complete evaluation of the liver requires overlapping these 2-cm near-field images across the entire length and breath of liver, which can be a time-consuming process [2].

Moreover, scanning becomes more difficult as the probe must be manipulated along a pivot point where the proximal shaft is fixed at the insertion port. The probe can be moved vertically in a cephalocaudal direction, but when it is moved laterally or medially, the shaft begins to pivot and the plane of view changes from a sagittal plane to an evermore oblique plane. With extreme pivoting, the plane of view may be closer to transverse than sagittal. This constantly changing plane of view can be disorienting, particularly to inexperienced observers. Constant reference to the orientation of the probe on the laparoscopic image can be helpful in attempting to overlap the imaging fields and obtain complete evaluation of the liver [2].

Before actually scanning, it is imperative to discuss with the clinicians and establish the information required by LUS. As patients are under general anesthesia and because of the high costs involved in an operating room setting, it is best to limit the amount of time used for LUS scanning to obtain the information required. It also is extremely beneficial to review any preoperative imaging, including previous ultrasound, CT, or MR imaging, before entering the operating room. Having these images directly available for consultation while in the operating room can help reduce overall study time and help focus the examination.

Operating room ergonomics

Optimal positioning of the monitors in relation to the probes can minimize difficulties and enhance the experience for LUS operators significantly. The monitors should be placed in a location that is natural for operators to manipulate the transducer while simultaneously viewing the monitors. Placing monitors in positions that force operators to

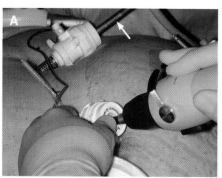
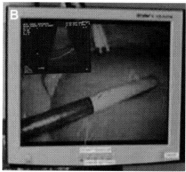

Fig. 5. Once inserted into the peritoneal cavity (*A*), the ultrasound probe (in the near field) must be watched continuously via the laparoscopic camera probe (*arrow*). Direct laparoscopic visualization of the ultrasound probe on the monitor (*B*) is essential at all times to avoid solid organ or vessel injury.

contort their bodies uncomfortably while manipulating the transducer should be avoided. The display monitors should be large enough and placed close enough to operators so that subtle abnormalities during scanning can be visualized easily.

Moreover, because operators view two screens simultaneously, a split screen (picture-in-picture) presentation using an electronic beam-splitting device is the optimal operating room scenario. These split-screen setups usually can adjust which real-time feed, the laparoscopic or ultrasound images, is displayed as the larger image and can be exchanged as needed. Displaying the laparoscopic and ultrasound images on the same monitor facilitates scanning and interpretation and at the same time reduces the risk of solid organ or vascular injury by the transducer.

Clinical applications of laparoscopic ultrasound

Laparoscopic ultrasound of the liver

As discussed previously, the liver is imaged best at a center frequency of 5 MHz, allowing for depth of penetration of 10 to 12 cm. Unlike standard IOUS, LUS takes considerably more time to scan the entire liver, as the near field is limited strictly by the length of the crystal. Complete scanning takes approximately 15 minutes with LUS versus 5 minutes with IOUS. Each survey of the liver should be done in an organized and systematic fashion, with the intention of overlapping each sequential imaging field completely so that the entire liver parenchyma is assessed (Fig. 6).

In a typical survey of the liver, a right subcostal port placement is used with direct and continuous visualization with the laparoscope from the standard periumbilical port. The LUS probe is passed as far cephalad as possible while the operator scans across the dome of the right lobe of the liver from left to right. The falciform ligament and ligamentum teres are barriers when imaging the left liver lobe via a right subcostal port and limit the medial extent of the sweep. Systematic scanning of the right and medial left lobes then are performed by withdrawing the probe approximately 2 cm in between overlapping sweeps across the liver.

Imaging of the left lateral segment requires either incision of the falciform ligament or switching ports between the laparoscopic and LUS probes or

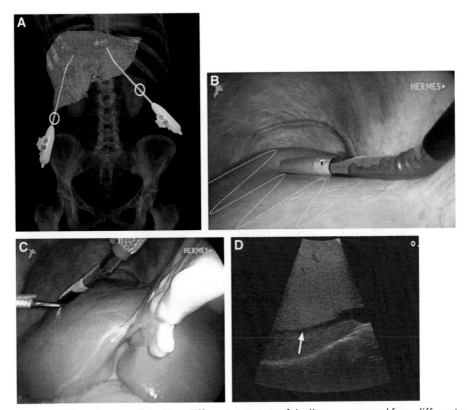

Fig. 6. For laparoscopic evaluation of the liver, different segments of the liver are accessed from different ports (*A*). Imaging is performed (*B*) with overlapping transverse scans (dotted lines). When imaging the hepatic dome (*C*), the probe must be positioned to the right of the fat-containing falciform ligament and flexed over the dome. In this way, structures, such as an accessory superior right hepatic vein (*D*) in segment VII (*arrow*), can be imaged.

forming a separate LUS probe insertion via a left subcostal port. Usually the periumbilical port is sufficient to access segments 1 to 3. Once the probe is in position at the dome of the left lateral segment, systematic scanning is performed again from left to right, with the falciform ligament again creating the barrier for the medial extent of the sweep.

The most common hepatic application of LUS is tumor staging. Laparoscopy often is used for preoperative staging of primary hepatic and metastatic tumors to optimally select candidates for resection (Fig. 7). Laparoscopy has proved superior to conventional preoperative imaging in staging of hepatocellular carcinoma, with more recent reports that laparoscopy with LUS provides superior information for the diagnosis and pretreatment staging of primary and metastatic hepatic tumors [6,12,13].

Obviously, deep liver tumor nodules cannot be detected with the laparoscope itself. LUS can reveal additional hepatic masses, metastatic lymphadenopathy, and vascular invasion not visualized on standard preoperative staging. Additional lesions disclosed on LUS generally are small, frequently less than 1 cm in diameter and, therefore, below the limit of resolution of most preoperative imaging modalities. Such findings can influence surgical decision-making and some studies have gone as far as to recommend routine use of LUS of the liver during all laparoscopic oncologic surgeries [13,14].

Other uses for LUS in the liver include accurate localization of tumors to specific lobes or segments and assessment of contiguous vascular and biliary structures. Invasions of bile ducts and the portal and hepatic venous system are well demonstrated.

Accessory vascular supply and venous drainage to and from the liver can influence the type and extent of resection to be performed greatly. LUS may be required to characterize vascular anastomoses after liver transplantation, to confirm patency of intrahepatic vessels, and to guide cautery on the liver capsule when these surface markers are used to guide deeper incisions. Replaced or accessory right and left hepatic arteries and accessory hepatic veins can be well demonstrated. LUS also can characterize lesions that are inconclusive on other imaging modalities, potentially influencing patient treatment. The ability to further characterize lesions using LUS may be most beneficial in determining benign abnormalities, such as focal fatty infiltration, focal areas of fatty sparing in a diffusely fatty liver, hemangiomas, or cysts from metastatic lesions.

Laparoscopic ultrasound of the gallbladder and bile ducts

The gallbladder and extrahepatic bile ducts usually can be imaged satisfactorily from a right subcostal port or from the periumbilical port. Also, from the left subcostal port, a so-called "Mickey Mouse" appearance of the ducts and adjacent hepatic artery is noted. The gallbladder is imaged best through the liver using a 5- or 7-MHz transducer. The extrahepatic bile ducts often are imaged best at 7 MHz though a compressed duodenum or gastric antrum, because near-field reverberation artifact limits sensitivity when the transducer is placed directly on the ducts. The distal-most portion of the CBD is visualized by imaging the head of the pancreas. Color flow

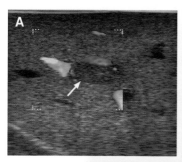

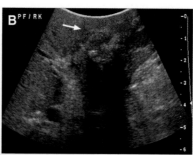

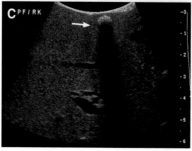

Fig. 7. LUS can be an effective tool for intraoperative oncologic staging. During a laparoscopic bowel resection for colon cancer (A), LUS identified an unexpected solitary hypoechoic lesion (arrow) in segment VII of the liver. LUS-guided biopsy confirmed metastatic tumor. LUS in a different patient who had mucinous colorectal metastases (B) demonstrated an ill-defined calcified mass arising in segment III of the liver (arrows). LUS at the time (C) also identified a calcified biopsy-proved metastatic subcapsular lesion (arrow) in segment V.

images are helpful for distinguishing the CBD from the portal vein and should be used routinely. Although the cystic duct usually is not well visualized on preoperative imaging, it can be identified routinely on LUS, including where it joins the CBD. This visualization can be helpful in identifying aberrant anatomy, such as a low insertion of the cystic duct into the CBD, which otherwise is unnoticed.

As laparoscopic cholecystectomy has become the standard of care in gallbladder disease, the use of LUS during these procedures is an increasing possibility. LUS can be a viable alternative to laparoscopic cholangiography. Common duct stones and strictures are visualized easily on LUS and it is recommended as the primary screening procedure for bile duct calculi because of its safety, speed, and cost-effectiveness [15]. Consequently, the routine use of laparoscopic cholangiography is not advised, because the yield of positive studies has proved low [16]. In the authors' experience, however, although LUS is available and efficacious, patients who have suspicious clinical, laboratory, or imaging findings for CBD abnormalities usually are referred for preoperative endoscopic retrograde cholangiopancreatography instead. As technology and experience with LUS advances, this could be an area for increased use in the future.

Further applications of LUS include oncologic staging of gallbladder and bile duct tumors, such as gallbladder carcinoma and cholangiocarcinoma (Fig. 8). The extent of invasion into the adjacent liver bed is difficult for surgeons to detect by inspection and palpation and can be portrayed well by IOUS [17]. Apart from identifying subtle liver metastasis (described previously), LUS can help define local extent of tumor and the involvement or sparing of ductal systems. LUS can help distinguish biliary sludge from intraluminal tumor with the use of targeted Doppler and color flow imaging. Moreover, benign strictures and malignant obstructions of the biliary tract can be defined further to help plan the type of biliary bypass procedure to be performed.

Laparoscopic ultrasound of the pancreas

The pancreas, from the head and uncinate process to the tail, can be imaged successfully at a 7-MHz frequency. The LUS approach to the pancreas is best through a right upper or left upper quadrant port, allowing the probe to be oriented along the long axis of the pancreas in a relatively transverse plane (Fig. 9). This allows for better orientation than attempting to image in the sagittal oblique plane across the short axis of the pancreas. The

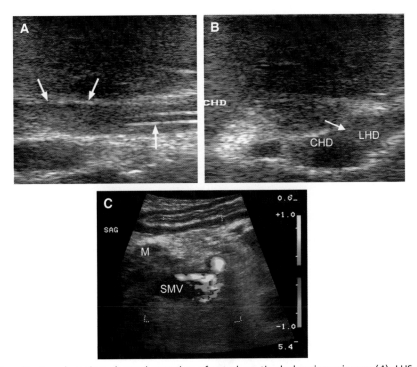

Fig. 8. In this patient undergoing planned resection of extrahepatic cholangiocarcinoma (*A*), LUS documented extent of involvement of the CBD (*angled arrows*). Tumor surrounds a previously placed biliary stent (*small vertical arrow*). Tumor extension (*B*) beyond the common hepatic duct (CHD) up into the left hepatic duct (LHD) (*arrow*) also was identified. In a different patient who had cholangiocarcinoma (*C*), LUS was used to localize the mass (M) and, using color flow, to confirm invasion of the superior mesenteric vein (SMV).

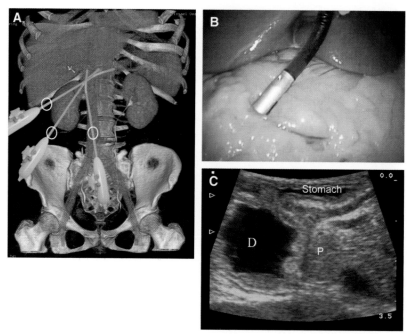

Fig. 9. For imaging the bile ducts and pancreatic head, probes (*A*) can be inserted in through right upper quadrant, right lower quadrant, or umbilical ports. The pancreatic body (*B*) can be imaged via a right subcostal port, typically imaged through the compressed stomach. When imaging the head (*C*) of the pancreas (*P*), the second part of the duodenum (*D*) is seen lateral to the head.

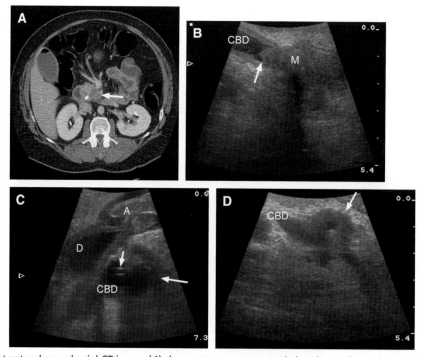

Fig. 10. Contrast-enhanced axial CT image (*A*) demonstrates a pancreatic head mass (*arrow*) encircling the CBD. At surgery, LUS (*B*) was used to localize the mass (*M*) and to document direct extension into the CBD (*arrow*). In a different patient (*C*), imaging through the compressed gastric antrum (*A*), an adenocarcinoma of the ampulla (*large arrow*) was identified in the head of the pancreas. Note the adjacent duodenum (*D*) and dilated CBD with a biliary stent (*small arrow*). LUS also showed (*D*) extension of the tumor (*arrow*), surrounding and extending into the CBD.

periumbilical port also can be useful in imaging the head/neck and uncinate process using a sagittal approach. Scanning can be performed directly on the pancreatic surface or through the overlying omentum. Occasionally, the lateral segment of the liver can provide an acoustic window to the pancreatic body and tail.

The main application for LUS in regard to pancreatic surgery is in conjunction with laparoscopic staging of pancreatic and periampullary tumors (Fig. 10). Although preoperative ultrasound, CT, and MR imaging can demonstrate vascular invasion or hepatic metastatic disease successfully, a significant number of patients who have advanced disease remain incompletely staged before surgery. Studies show the improved staging of pancreatic and perimpullary tumors by laparoscopy with LUS versus standard preoperative imaging methods [7,18].

LUS of the pancreas also is described as a sensitive and successful method in localizing islet cell tumors (Fig. 11) [19,20]. This method may be important particularly for small lesions localized to the body or tail of the pancreas, because laparoscopic partial pancreatic resections can be performed. Laparoscopy with LUS is reported to contribute significantly to the differential diagnosis of pancreatic cystic neoplasms [21,22], helping delineate serous microcystic adenomas, mucinous cystadenomas, or cystadenocarcinomas and intraductal papillary mucinous neoplasms of the pancreas (Fig. 12). LUS imaging also can help identify the extent of pseudocysts and pancreatic ductal abnormalities in patients who have pancreatitis. Transgastric LUS imaging can be used to facilitate laparoscopic cystgastrostomy.

Other applications

As more and more surgical procedures move to laparoscopic approaches, the possible applications for LUS continue to increase. There are reports of improved localization of intra-abdominal tumors using LUS during planned laparoscopic resections. For example, LUS shows improved localization of adrenal tumors by defining the relationship to adjacent structures and providing confirmation that larger tumors are amenable to laparoscopic resection [23]. Reports of LUS use in gynecologic surgery also are increasing, with studies describing improved laparoscopic ovarian tumor localization and staging [24] and management of ovarian cysts and adnexal masses [25]. LUS also is used to evaluate ureteral location and function during

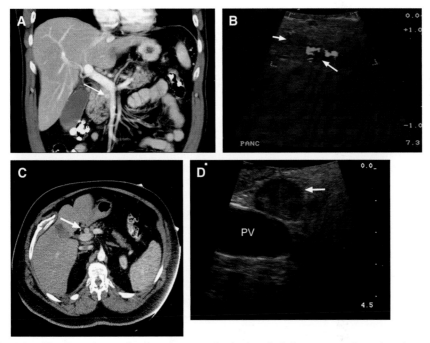

Fig. 11. After identification of a small enhancing mass in the head of the pancreas lateral to the superior mesenteric vein (*arrow*) on a contrast-enhanced CT scan (*A*), LUS (*B*) was performed to confirm and characterize the mass (*small arrow*) and depict proximity of the mass to the adjacent superior mesenteric vein (*large arrow*). Based on the LUS findings, laparoscopy was converted to an open procedure and resection revealed an islet cell tumor. In another patient, a 3-mm enhancing lesion (*C*) was identified on a contrast-enhanced CT scan (*arrow*). LUS (*D*) was used to localize the lesion (*arrow*) to show absence of portal vein (PV) invasion and to guide surgical resection, which showed a nonfunctioning insulinoma.

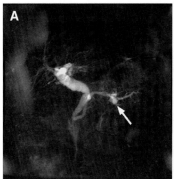
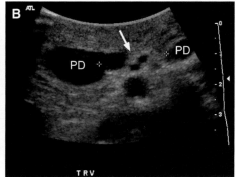

Fig. 12. After identification of a cystic mass (*A*) in the body of the pancreas on this coronal T2-weighted magnetic resonance cholangiopancreatography image (*arrow*), LUS (*B*) was used to localize the mass (*arrow*) and guide the resection. Note the dilated pancreatic ducts (PD) proximal and distal to the mass. Pathology confirmed that this was an intraductal papillary mucinous neoplasm.

laparoscopic gynecologic surgery to help lower the incidence of intraoperative ureteral complications [26]. The full and complete use of LUS remains to be seen.

Biopsy and percutaneous ablation guidance

Superficial and larger deep tumors within organs can be biopsied readily under direct laparoscopic visualization or with LUS assistance (Fig. 13). Traditional LUS-guided biopsies require placing the transducer over the site to be biopsied followed by percutaneous insertion of a long needle through the abdominal wall down to the level of the transducer. This technique can make small, deep lesions difficult to biopsy because of the considerable distances between the needle insertion in the anterior abdominal wall and the location of the LUS probe. When lesions are located in deep positions, it may be necessary to vent some gas from the peritoneal cavity once the transducer is placed on the biopsy

site to minimize the distance. Newer-generation laparoscopic probes, however, are designed with puncture and biopsy guides, making small, deep lesions easier to biopsy under LUS guidance.

LUS also has the potential to guide minimally invasive tumor ablations, although experience thus far is limited. Minimally invasive oncology therapies technology, such as radiofrequency ablation, microwave ablation, and cryosurgery, continue to be developed and used. With the improved tumor localization provided by LUS, evolution to LUS-guided minimally invasive therapies is a logical next step.

Summary

As more open surgical procedures move to laparoscopic approaches, the demand for LUS continues to increase. New improvements in technology and equipment already have advanced LUS from its experimental beginnings to the point of routine

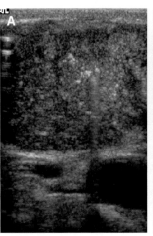
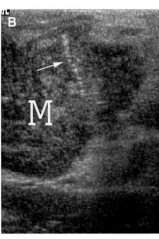

Fig. 13. (*A,B*) A percutaneous needle (*arrow*) is inserted into a hypoechoic pancreatic mass (M) adjacent to the transducer for LUS-guided pancreas biopsy. Although adenocarcinoma was suspected from preoperative imaging studies, pathology revealed lymphocytic sclerosing pancreatitis.

clinical applications. Applications in the liver, pancreas, gallbladder, and biliary tree are described, with further applications in gynecologic surgery also reported. The applications in LUS-guided biopsies and minimally invasive therapies remain to be perfected. An operator learning curve remains, however, and mastery of LUS requires familiarity with the special equipment and scanning techniques. But as technology and the widespread use continue to advance, the full range and importance of LUS applications no doubt will increase.

References

[1] Kane RA, Hughs LA, Cua EJ, et al. The impact of intraoperative ultrasonography on surgery for liver neoplasms. J Ultrasound Med 1994;13:1–6.

[2] Kane RA. Laparoscopic ultrasound. In: Kane RA, editor. Intraoperative, laparoscopic, and endoluminal ultrasound. Philadelphia: Churchill Livingstone; 1999. p. 90–105.

[3] Ascher SM, Evans SRT, Goldberg JA, et al. Intraoperative bile duct sonography during laparoscopic cholecystectomy: experience with a 12.5 MHz catheter based US probe. Radiology 1992; 185:493–6.

[4] Yamamoto M, Stiegmann GV, Durham J, et al. Laparoscopy-guided intracorporeal ultrasound accurately delineates hepatobiliary anatomy. Surg Endosc 1993;7:325–30.

[5] Goletti O, Celona G, Galatioto C, et al. Is laparoscopic sonography a reliable and sensitive procedure for staging colorectal cancer? A comparative study. Surg Endosc 1998;12:1236–41.

[6] Montorsi M, Santambrogio R, Bianchi P, et al. Laparoscopy with laparoscopic ultrasound for pretreatment staging of hepatocellular carcinoma: a prospective study. J Gastrointest Surg 2001;5:312–5.

[7] Doran HE, Bosonnet L, Connor S, et al. Laparoscopy and laparoscopic ultrasound in the evaluation of pancreatic and periampullary tumours. Dig Surg 2004;21:305–13.

[8] Vollmer CM, Drebin JA, Middleton WD, et al. Utility of staging laparoscopy in subsets of peripancreatic and biliary malignancies. Ann Surg 2002;235:1–7.

[9] Yamakawa K, Naito S, Azuma K, et al. Laparoscopic diagnosis of the intra-abdominal organs. Jpn J Gastroenterol 1958;55:741–7.

[10] Yamakawa K, Yoshioka A, Shimizu K, et al. Laparoechography: an ultrasonic diagnosis under laparoscopic observation. Jpn Med Ultrasonics 1964;2:26.

[11] Fornari F, Civardi G, Cavanna L, et al. Laparoscopic ultrasonography in the study of liver diseases. Preliminary results. Surg Endosc 1989; 3:33–7.

[12] Foroutani A, Garland AM, Berber E, et al. Laparoscopic ultrasound vs triphasic computed tomography for detecting liver tumors. Arch Surg 2000; 135:933–8.

[13] Thaler K, Kanneganti S, Khajanchee Y, et al. The evolving role of staging laparoscopy in the treatment of colorectal hepatic metastasis. Arch Surg 2005;140:727–34.

[14] Milsom JW, Jerby BL, Kessler H, et al. Prospective, blinded comparison of laparoscopic ultrasonography vs. contrast-enhanced computerized tomography for liver assessment in patients undergoing colorectal carcinoma surgery. Dis Colon Rectum 2000;43:44–9.

[15] Machi J, Tateishi T, Oishi AJ, et al. Laparoscopic ultrasonography versus operative cholangiography during laparoscopic cholecystectomy: review of the literature and a comparison with open intraoperative ultrasonography. J Am Coll Surg 1999;188:360–7.

[16] Rothlin MA, Schlumpf R, Largiader F. Laparoscopic sonography. Arch Surg 1994;129: 694–700.

[17] Azuma T, Yoshikawa T, Ariada T, et al. Intraoperative evaluation of the depth of invasion of gallbladder cancer. Am J Surg 1999;178:381–4.

[18] Taylor AM, Roberts SA, Manson JM. Experience with laparoscopic ultrasonography for defining tumour resectability in carcinoma of the pancreatic head and periampullary region. Br J Surg 2001;88:1077–83.

[19] Lo CY, Lo CM, Fan ST. Role of laparoscopic ultrasonography in intraoperative localization of pancreatic insulinoma. Surg Endosc 2000;14: 1131–5.

[20] Ishihara M, Kanbe M, Okamoto T, et al. Laparoscopic ultrasonography for resection of insulinomas. Surgery 2001;130:1086–91.

[21] Schachter PP, Avni Y, Gvirz G, et al. The impact of laparoscopy and laparoscopic ultrasound on the management of pancreatic cystic lesions. Arch Surg 2000;135:260–4.

[22] Schachter PP, Shimonov M, Czerniak A. The role of laparoscopy and laparoscopic ultrasound in the diagnosis of cystic lesions of the pancreas. Gastrointest Endosc Clin North Am 2002;12: 759–67.

[23] Brunt LM, Bennett HF, Teefey SA, et al. Laparoscopic ultrasound imaging of adrenal tumors during laparoscopic adrenalectomy. Am J Surg 1999;178:490–5.

[24] Helin HL, Kirkinen P. Laparoscopic ultrasonography during conservative ovarian surgery. Surg Endosc 2000;14:161–3.

[25] Noyan V, Tiras MB, Oktem M, et al. Laparoscopic ultrasonography in the management of ovarian cysts. Gynecol Obstet Invest 2005;60:63–6.

[26] Helin-Martikainen HL, Kirkinen P. Ultrasonography of the ureter during laparoscopic gynecological surgery. Ultrasound Obstet Gynecol 1997; 9:414–8.

ELSEVIER
SAUNDERS

ULTRASOUND
CLINICS

Ultrasound Clin 1 (2006) 559–565

Index

Note: Page numbers of article titles are in **boldface** type.

1556-858X/06/$ – see front matter © 2006 Elsevier Inc. All rights reserved.
ultrasound.theclinics.com

doi:10.1016/S1556-858X(06)00056-9